BY A. DUGAN AND THE EDITORS OF CONSUMER GUIDE®

New Quick, Easy Way To
Flatten Your Stomach
For Men Over 40

CONTENTS

Louis Weber, President
Publications International, Ltd.
3841 West Oakton Street
Skokie, Illinois 60076

Permission is never granted for commercial purposes.

Manufactured in the United States of America
10 9 8 7 6 5 4 3 2

ISBN: 0-88176-249-0

Design: Inez Smith
Photography: Sam Griffith Studios
Model: Chuck Swenson

THE FLATTEN YOUR STOMACH PROGRAM

Nothing "makes the man" more than a trim physique. And men tend to have even greater appeal as they mature—particularly if they are strong and fit. A trim body—with a firm, flat stomach—tells the world that you have taken command of your health and fitness. Fitness is more important after 40 than at any other time in life, for this is when the aging process tends to begin. But you can slow down, stop, and even reverse many of the physical effects associated with aging. You need not invest a great deal of time, money, and exhaustive effort. All it takes is a good offensive game plan—like the fitness plan in this book.

The Flatten Your Stomach Program is a fast, effective exercise plan designed especially for men over 40. It concentrates on the stomach muscles, which are the first to age, slacken, and accumulate fat—suggesting a loss of youth and vigor. Now you can regain and maintain that trim, youthful look. With the Flatten Your Stomach Program, you can tone and firm your muscles, lower your body fat, and build the strength and endurance you need to lead a healthy, vigorous life.

GETTING ON THE RIGHT TRACK

If you have been exercising and watching what you eat, but you are still out of shape, you've been working on the wrong program. Too often, men do only sit-ups and toe-touches, which exercise only one muscle area. If you do this, your stomach may be hard, but it may still bulge because you are overdeveloping one set of muscles at the expense of the others. That is why you need a balanced program to trim and tone all the muscle layers that mold and shape the stomach area.

The Flatten Your Stomach Program works because it exercises all four sets of muscles in the stomach area. It also alternates dense muscle contractions with stretching exercises so that there is a complete balance in strength and tone of all the stomach muscles. These muscles usually respond rapidly to a well-designed exercise plan. After just a few weeks with the Flatten Your Stomach Program, you'll be amazed at the difference in the way you look and feel.

FOLLOWING THE PROGRAM

The Flatten Your Stomach Program consists of warm up exercises, muscle toning exercises for the stomach area, and cool down exercises. The stomach flattening exercises are divided into three levels: Beginning, Intermediate, and Advanced. Always start your workout with the Warm Up and end it with the Cool Down, regardless of what level you are working on in the stomach flattening exercises.

To get the most out of the workout, you need to put some effort into preparing for it. That means you must warm up properly. The warm up helps your body ease into more vigorous activity and lessens your chances of being injured. A good warm up raises your body's internal temperature and stimulates the movement of oxygen and blood in the body. The warm up conditions the heart muscle and increases breathing in order to supply more oxygen to the muscles. The warm up also contains stretches to condition and lengthen the ligaments and tendons around the joints. Do the stretching movements slowly, in a controlled fashion. Avoid fast, jerky movements which could result in injury to the joints or tearing of the muscle fibers.

Toward the end of the workout, you will notice that your heart and lungs are working at a higher rate than usual. This is because exercise has increased the body's need for oxygen. Even after you have stopped exercising, the need for extra oxygen continues for several minutes. This is why the cool down is important. The cool down helps the muscles get rid of built-up waste products (lactic acid), thus reducing muscle stiffness the next day. The cool down also returns the circulation to the pre-exercise state (thereby preventing light-headedness or dizziness) and gradually returns breathing to normal. You should feel relaxed but invigorated after doing the cool down exercises.

HOW TO USE THE PROGRAM

No matter what your present level of fitness may be, start with the Beginning Program. Then gradually work your way up through to the Intermediate and Advanced Programs. The number of times you should repeat each exercise is indicated in the exercise instructions. If the number of repetitions indicated seems too difficult, do fewer repetitions to start. You can gradually add more repetitions as you build up strength. Never push yourself to the point of strain or injury. Start slowly and work at a pace that is comfortable for you.

Here are guidelines for working your way through the program, from the beginning level up through the intermediate and advanced levels.

Beginning Program

When you first start this exercise program, your workout should consist of the following exercises:
1. Do all of the exercises in the Warm Up section.
2. Do 6 exercises of your choice from the Beginning Program, as follows:
   2 standing exercises;
   2 kneeling exercises;
   2 exercises lying on the back or sitting.
3. Do all of the exercises in the Cool Down section.
As your strength and endurance increases, gradually add more exercises each week until you can easily complete all the exercises in the Beginning Program (in addition to the Warm Up and Cool Down). As you increase the number of exercises, you may wish to reduce the number of repetitions for each exercise for a while. Then gradually add repetitions again until you are doing all of the exercises in the Beginning Program at the number of repetitions indicated in the instructions.

Intermediate Program

When the entire Beginning Program becomes comfortable and easy to do (usually after about 4 to 6 weeks), start the Intermediate Program as follows:
1. Do all of the exercises in the Warm Up section.
2. Do 12 exercises of your choice from the Intermediate Program, as follows:
   4 standing exercises;
   8 exercises lying on the back or sitting.
3. Do all of the exercises in the Cool Down section.
Then gradually add more exercises each week until you can easily complete all of the exercises in the Intermediate Program at the number of repetitions indicated in the instructions (in addition to the Warm Up and Cool Down).

Advanced Program

When the entire Intermediate Program becomes easy for you, go on to the Advanced Program, as follows:
1. Do all of the exercises in the Warm Up section.
2. Do 12 exercises of your choice from the Advanced Program as follows:
   4 standing exercises;
   8 exercises kneeling, lying on the back, or sitting.
3. Do all of the exercises in the Cool Down section.
Gradually add exercises each week until you are doing all of the exercises in the Advanced Program at the number of repetitions indicated in the instructions (along with the Warm Up and Cool Down). You can continue to work on the Advanced Program indefinitely to maintain the fitness level you have achieved.

In the beginning, your workout may take about 20 minutes to complete, since you will be doing fewer exercises. As you add more exercises, the workout should last about 40 minutes to receive the most benefit from the program.

When you first begin the Flatten Your Stomach Program, it is recommended that you work out 3 days a week, alternating exercise days with days of rest. As you advance, work up to exercising 5 days a week. Establish a routine and stick to it. Make exercise an essential part of your life.

If you are off the program for any length of time, go back and start with the Beginning Program, and again work up slowly to the Advanced Program. Remember, it takes only 72 hours for the body to start losing its strength and endurance! So once you get started, keep with it.

TRAINING HEART RATES*
To Determine the Conditioning Effects of Exercise

Age	Beats in 10 seconds		Beats in 1 minute	
	Minimum 70%	Maximum 85%	Minimum 70%	Maximum 85%
40	21	26	126	156
45	21	25	126	150
50	20	24	120	144
55	19	23	114	138
60	19	23	114	138
65	18	22	108	132
70	17	21	102	126
75	17	20	102	120

These figures are averages for healthy individuals. For exact figures for yourself, ask your doctor. If your age falls between the ages shown in the chart, follow the averages for the age higher than your own age. Note that with training, cardiovascular efficiency and strength changes very little with aging.

THE TRAINING RANGE

The Warm Up and the first group of standing exercises in each program are aerobic exercises. That means that they are conditioning the heart and lungs, as well as the stomach muscles. By working these muscles in this way, you are increasing your heart rate, strengthening the heart muscle, burning off excess fat, and raising the internal body temperature to prepare for the rest of the workout. One of the major benefits of this program is its emphasis on the "training effect" of exercise. This term refers to the improved physical capacity developed by regular aerobic exercise, which increases the body's strength and efficiency.

Each person's response to exercise is different. Therefore, it is important that you carefully monitor your body's responses during your workout. You monitor the heart by taking the pulse. A normal pulse (heart rate) in adults ranges between 60 and 80 beats per minute. Regular exercise may lower the resting pulse rate. Checking your pulse during exercise tells you how your body is responding to the exercise and tells you the conditioning you are receiving from the training part of the program.

When you exercise, your heart should be beating at 70 to 85 percent of its maximum rate for your age group. This 70 to 85 percent of your maximum heart rate is called the "training range" or "target heart rate zone." If your heart rate is below 70 percent during exercise, you're not sufficiently challenging your heart and circulatory system. If it is above 85 percent, you're challenging it too much, and you should pause briefly to rest until the heart rate returns to within 70 to 85 percent of your maximum heart rate.

To find out if you're in the "training range," stop after the warm up, take your pulse for 10 seconds and compare it with the chart in this section. Multiply this number by 6 to get the number of beats per minute. If your heart rate is within the recommended training range, continue working. Then take the pulse again 15 to 20 minutes later.

Notice that the training heart rate will improve as you advance through the program. However, do *not* try to attain the training heart rate when you first start the program, and do *not* try to work up to it too quickly. Take the resting heart rate before beginning exercise and again 10 minutes after finishing the workout. The pulse should return to normal (the approximate beginning resting heart rate) by that time.

The pulse is usually taken:
1. At the radial artery, which is in the wrist just below the base of the thumb.
2. At the carotid artery, which is in the side

of the neck underneath the jaw bone.
3. At the inside of the elbow, just above the skin crease.

To take your pulse at the radial artery, place your first two fingers on the inside of your wrist just below your thumb. Count the number of beats for 10 seconds. Then multiply that number by 6 to determine your pulse rate per minute.

Improving your "training range" increases endurance and metabolic rate. The basal metabolic rate decreases slightly but steadily throughout life. That means the rate at which we use energy slows down, and we are burning calories less efficiently in our daily routines. Physical activity increases the basal metabolic rate. And once it is raised, it takes several hours to return to the normal state. This means that the body continues to burn extra calories even after you stop exercising. Muscle tissue uses up more energy than body fat, so most males are blessed with faster basal metabolic rates than are females since males have a higher percentage of muscle mass.

COMBINE EXERCISE WITH GOOD NUTRITION

Along with this exercise program, watch what you eat. Select a variety of foods from each of the four basic food groups, and eat moderate portions. The diet recommended by the American Heart Association for promoting optimal health is well balanced and nutritious. The caloric content for men over 40 should be around 2,000 calories per day. For those who want to lose weight, it should be about 1,500 calories per day. Fat intake should be limited to approximately 30 percent of the calories per day, with the remainder of the nutrient intake divided between proteins and carbohydrates. It is also important to limit your intake of sugar, starch, and salt.

Diet is one of the most important controlling factors in the constant growth and repair of the body. While a good diet can't guarantee that you will be in good health, you can't be in the best of health *unless* you live on a good diet. The study of nutrition and its relation to maintaining good health should be a prime consideration throughout life.

HYPERTENSION – WHAT IS IT?

First, the word does not mean being excessively tense or nervous. *Hypertension* is the medical term for high blood pressure. Blood pressure is a variable and can change from minute to minute, with change in body position, exercise, degree of tension, body fluid levels, caffeine, foods, weight, smoking, and sleep.

Blood pressure is recorded by measuring the systolic and diastolic pressure as follows: 120/80 (systolic/diastolic). *Systolic* pressure is the blood pressure in the arteries when the heart is pumping blood. *Diastolic* pressure is the pressure in the arteries when the heart is filling with blood for the next beat. Normal blood pressure is defined as below 140/90. Blood pressure above 150/100 is considered hypertension. Blood pressures falling between these two are called borderline hypertension and may or may not require treatment.

A person with hypertension may not even know it, because, in the early stages, there are few if any symptoms. An early morning headache, flushing of the face, dizziness, nosebleeds, blurred vision, and swings of high and normal pressure may give some indication of hypertension. This does not mean the vital organs are being affected. However, when the body is affected by high blood pressure, the walls of the arteries become more rigid, and the heart must work extra hard to pump blood through small openings. If left untreated, complications may eventually develop. High blood pressure can result in heart disease, kidney disease, or stroke. High blood pressure cannot be cured, but it can be controlled. Medication and lifestyle changes are usually recommended by your doctor. To control or avoid high blood pressure, keep these guidelines in mind:

- Keep your weight down.
- Exercise regularly.
- Reduce salt intake.
- Reduce the amount of fat in your diet.
- Get adequate relaxation.
- Don't smoke.
- Have your blood pressure checked frequently, since hypertension is more likely to occur after the age of 40.

OH, MY ACHING BACK!

A weak back and weak stomach muscles go hand in hand. If the stomach muscles are weak, the internal organs slip and press against the abdominal wall. As the organs progressively slip, the muscles progressively weaken and the stomach protrudes even more. The situation is complicated by the fact that a sagging waistline throws the body posture out of kilter. Any excess weight causes the pelvis to drop in front and rise in back, especially when the stomach muscles are too weak to hold the pelvis in place. Due to misalignment of the pelvis, the part of the spinal column that is attached to the pelvis rotates forward causing a "swayback." The sway causes the vertebrae of the spine to squeeze together, which in turn puts pressure on the nerves in the area. The result is low back pain. There are numerous other reasons for back pain, such as wearing away of the discs, arthritis, herniated disc, injury, or torn muscles and ligaments. Back pain has plagued man since the beginning of time, and it has affected people from all walks of life and every profession. There have been many suggested "cures." But the most widely prescribed remedy is this: exercise properly to strengthen the stomach and back muscles. Therefore, an added benefit of the Flatten Your Stomach Program is the conditioning effect it will have on your back.

PROGRAM GUIDELINES

1. It is recommended that you consult your doctor before beginning this or any other exercise program.

2. If you have not been exercising regularly or if you have a medical history that would limit activity, consult your doctor as to which exercises in this program are best for you.

3. Wear comfortable clothing so that your movements are not restricted.

4. Wear an athletic shoe or a firm support shoe that will help absorb shock to the ankles, knees, and back.

5. While exercising, breathe normally. Do not hold the breath or use controlled or forced breathing.

6. Avoid dizziness by pausing briefly before changing direction.

7. Stop exercising if you feel dizzy or nauseated.

8. Start slowly, doing the number of repetitions indicated in the exercise instructions (or fewer). Then work up gradually to more repetitions.

9. Eat only in moderation during the two hours before you exercise; otherwise nausea could occur.

10. Try to do the program at the same time each day you work out so that you establish a routine. The time of day you exercise is not important. Choose a time that's best for you, and stick to your routine.

11. Do not expect to be of equal strength or vigor each day. Some days you may be more up to it.

12. Do not overstress yourself. Work to the point of fatigue—*not* to the point of exhaustion, strain, or injury.

13. Monitor your heart by checking your pulse throughout the program. Also watch for signs of stress, strain, or injury.

14. Some soreness can be expected at first since you are using muscles you may not have exercised for some time.

15. Supplement this program with as much recreational physical activity as possible, such as golf, swimming, or walking.

16. Form is critical. Try to do the exercises exactly as indicated.

17. Use a mat, thick carpet, or folded towel when doing the floor exercises to avoid rubbing or irritation to the coccyx (tailbone).

18. Notice that some of the exercises instruct you to keep the feet flat (not pointed). The purpose of this is to condition and lengthen the hamstring muscles in the backs of the legs. It also makes the pull on the stomach muscles stronger.

19. Notice that some exercises instruct you to clasp your hands behind the head (*not* behind the neck). This is to prevent the head from bobbing, which would place undue stress on the neck.

EXERCISE!

Medical authorities believe that exercise may be the single most effective way to improve the length and the quality of life. We were designed to be active. So go to it! No matter what shape you are in now or what age you are, you can improve and achieve dramatic results through exercise. You can look and feel better than you ever have before.

WARM UP

REACH AND STRETCH

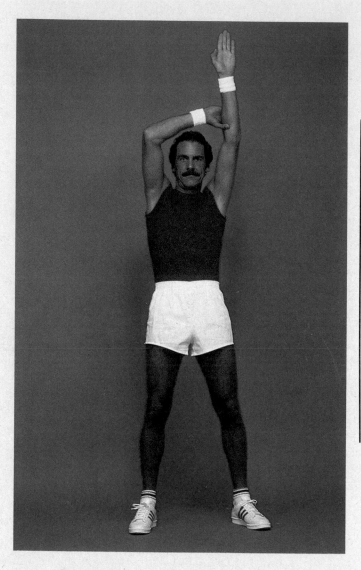

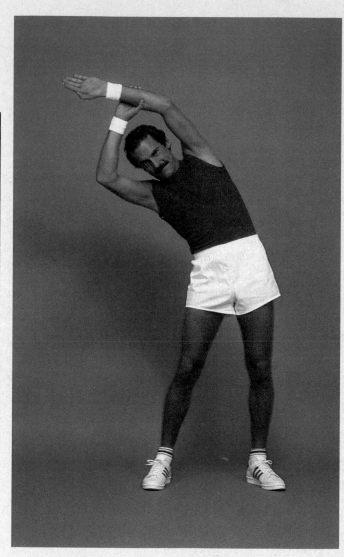

1 Stand with the feet wide apart, left arm extended straight up, right hand clasping the left arm.

2 Slowly pull the left arm to the right, bending to the side from the waist. Hold for 5 counts. Return to the starting position. Repeat, pulling the right arm to the left. Do 3 to 5 times, alternating left and right.

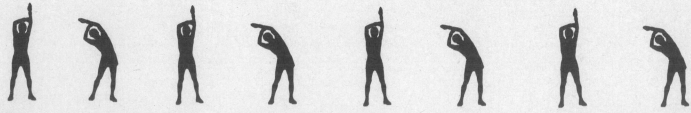

PULL AND STRETCH

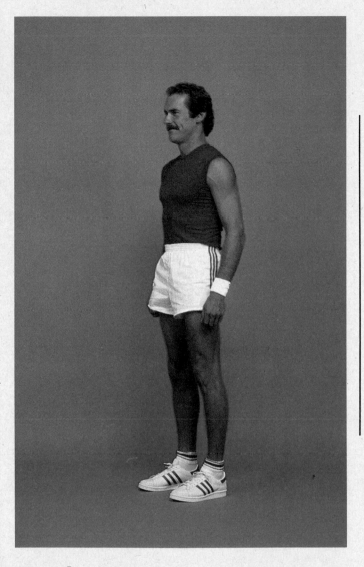

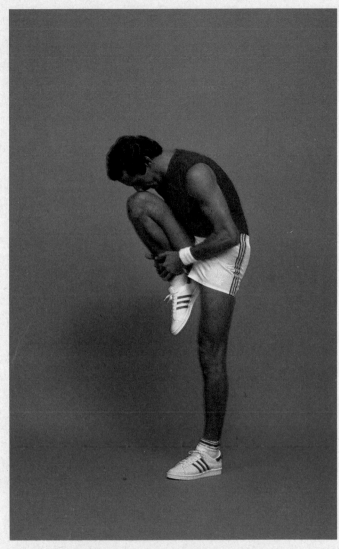

1 Stand with the feet slightly apart, arms at the sides.

2 Raise the right knee to the chest, clasping the knee with both hands. Pull the knee up as high as possible, and press the head down toward the knee. Hold for 5 counts. Return to the starting position. Repeat with the left knee. Do 3 to 5 times, alternating right and left.

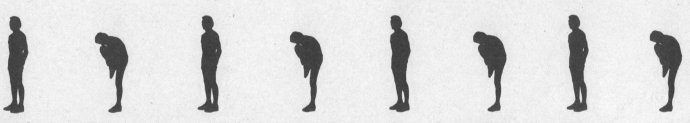

CONDITIONING STRETCH

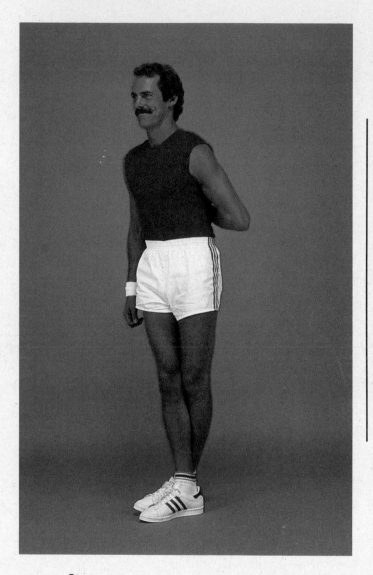

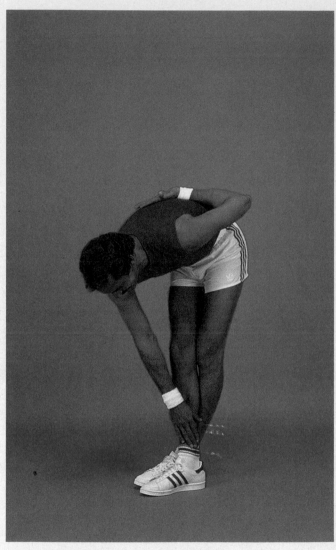

1 Stand with the right leg crossed in front of the left, right arm at the side. Bend the left arm up in back, reaching up the back as far as possible.

2 Slowly bend down and touch the right hand to the right ankle. Hold for 5 counts. Return to the starting position. Do 3 to 5 times. Then reverse the arm and leg positions, and touch the left hand to the left ankle 3 to 5 times.

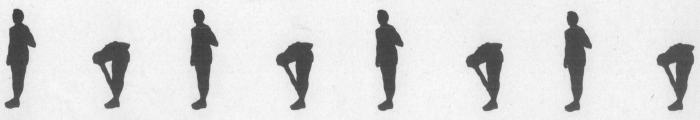

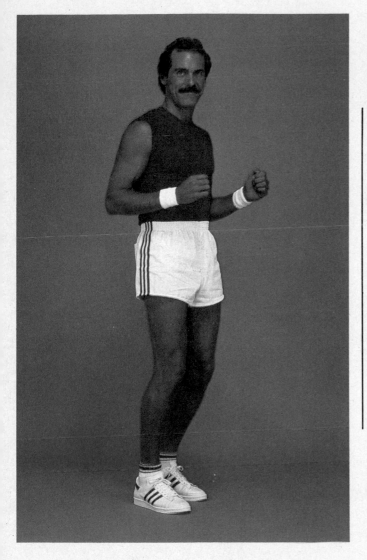

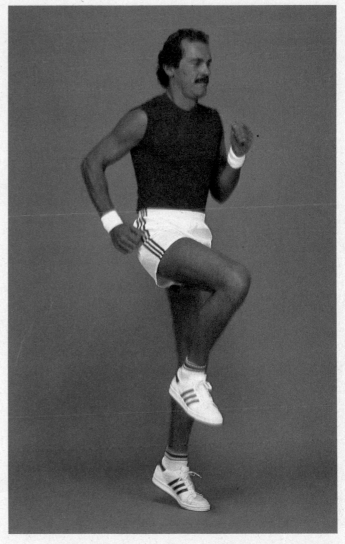

1 Stand with the feet slightly apart, knees slightly bent, arms bent at waist height.

2 Run in place. Start with 1 minute and gradually advance to 3 minutes. You may slowly work yourself up to 12 minutes (depending on your body conditioning).

This is an aerobic exercise to strengthen and condition the heart, as well as to increase the metabolic rate, which helps regulate weight.

Check your pulse immediately afterward. Consult the chart in the introduction to this book to see if you are attaining your correct "target heart rate" range.

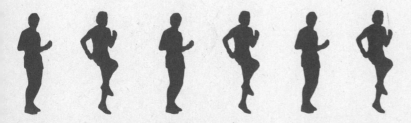

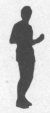

BEGINNING PROGRAM

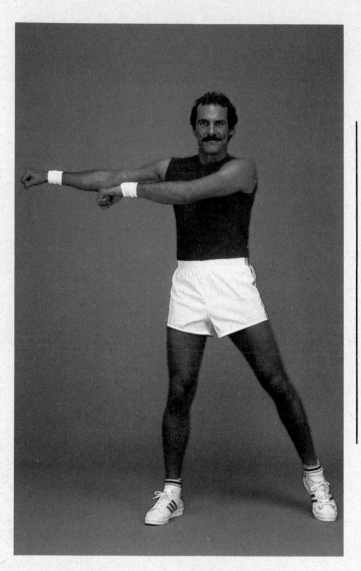

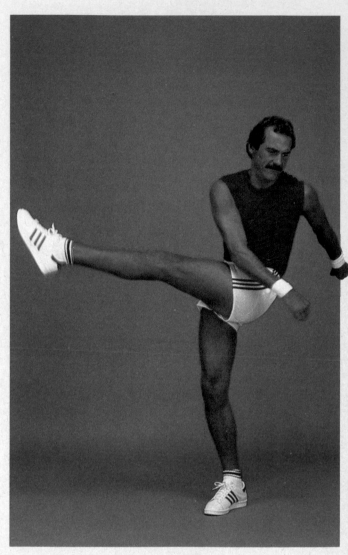

1 Stand with the weight on the right leg, left leg to the side with the weight on the toes, both arms extended to the right at chest height, hands in fists.

2 Swing the left leg up to the right. At the same time, swing both arms down toward the left hip. Return to the starting position. Do 8 times with each leg.

SIDE KICK

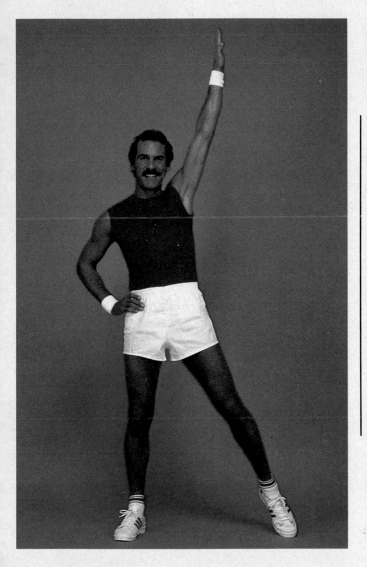

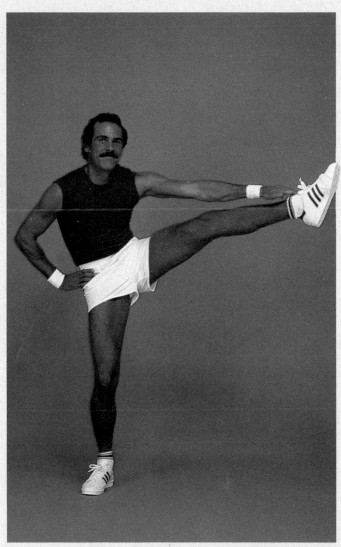

1 Stand with the weight on the right leg, left leg to the side with the weight on the toes, right hand on the hip, left arm extended up.

2 Raise the left leg up to the side as high as possible, and touch the left hand to the left leg. Return to the starting position. Do 8 times with each leg.

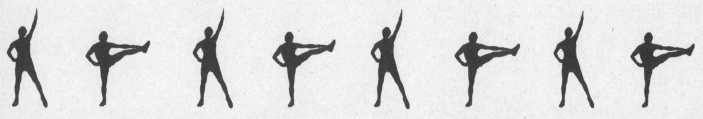

ROTATE

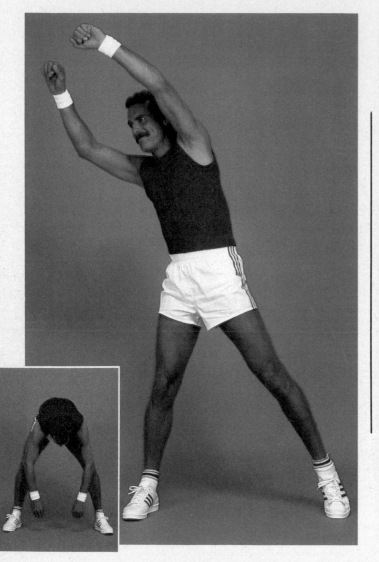

1 Stand with the knees bent, torso leaning over the floor, both arms hanging toward the floor in a relaxed position.

2 Straightening the knees, swing both arms up to the right.

3 Continue in a circular motion, swinging the arms up overhead, down to the left, and back down to the starting position. Do 8 circles to the right, and 8 to the left.

Great for the back, waistline, and stomach.

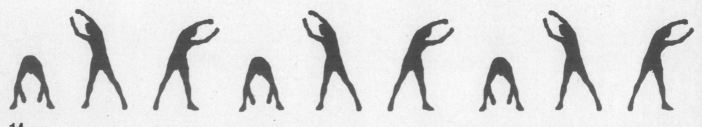

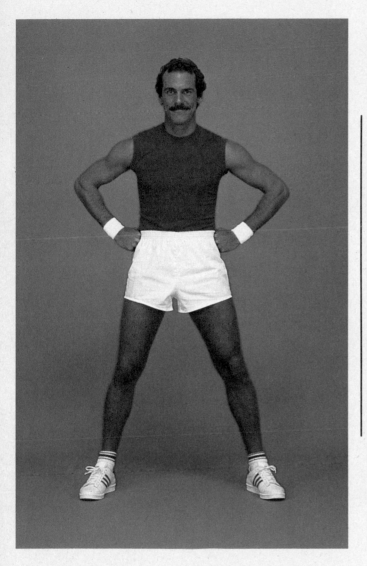

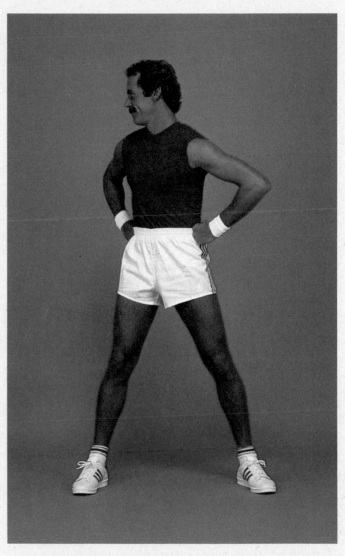

1 Stand with the feet wide apart, toes forward, hands on the hips.

2 Twist the torso to the right, turning the head with the twist. Then twist to the left. Do 10 times, alternating right and left.

Do this exercise slowly and smoothly. Avoid quick, jerking movements, which could cause back strain. Do not twist any farther than is comfortable for the back and neck.

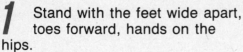

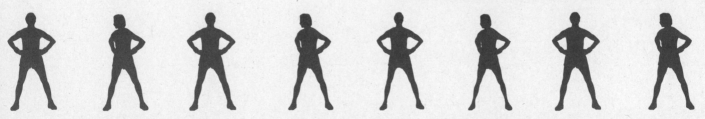

LEAN AND SLIM

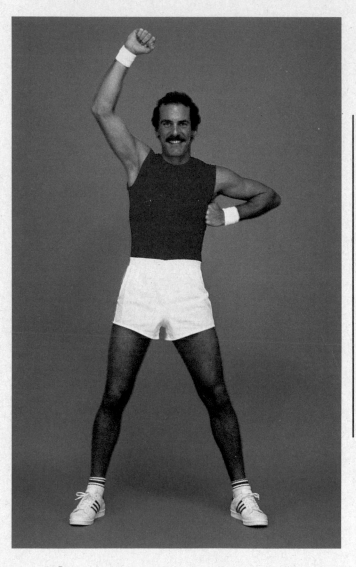

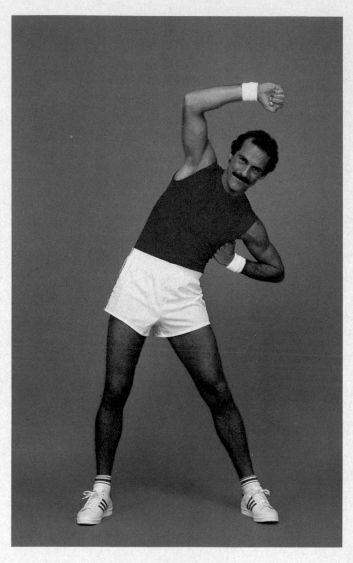

1 Stand with the feet wide apart, hands in fists, left hand pressing into the armpit, right arm in an arc overhead.

2 Keeping the left arm in position, bend to the left side, pressing the right arm to the left. Return to the starting position. Do 10 times to each side.

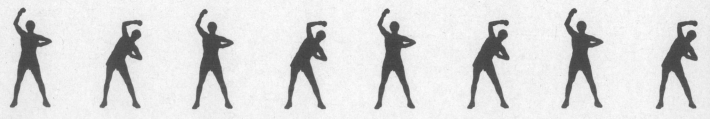

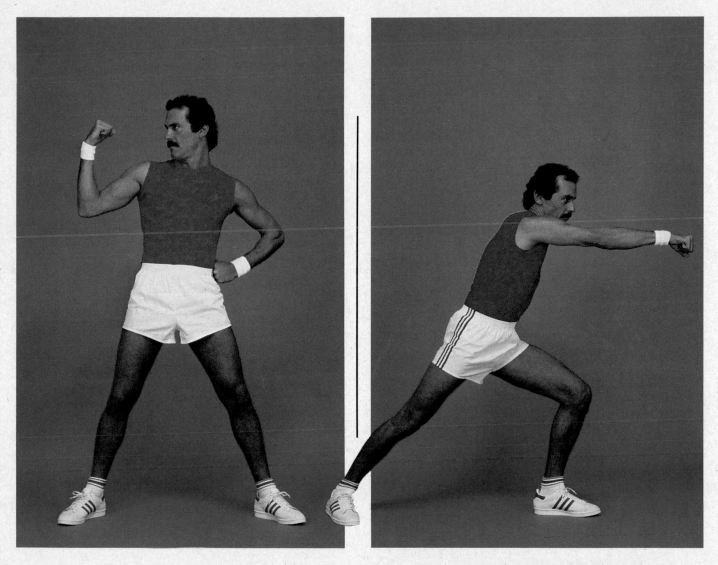

1 Stand with the feet wide apart, knees slightly bent, left hand on the hip, right arm bent up at the side with the hand in a fist.

2 Bend the left knee, and turn toward the left, pivoting on the right foot. Extend the right arm to the left in a jabbing motion. Return to the starting position. Do 10 times to each side.

TRIMMER

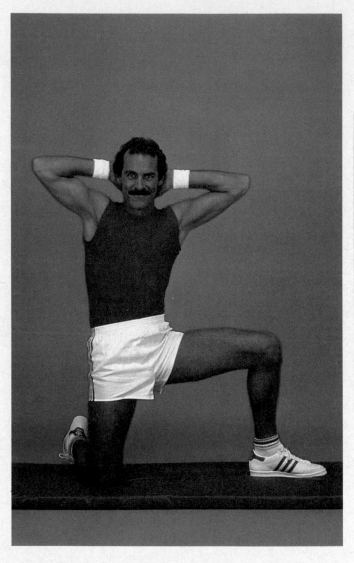

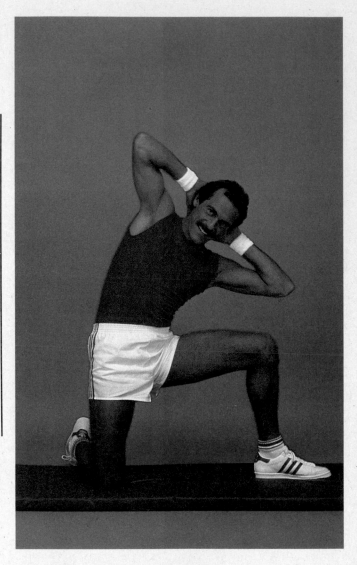

1 Kneel on the right knee, left leg bent to the side with the foot on the floor, hands clasped behind the head.

2 Bend to the side, and try to touch the left elbow to the left knee. Return to the starting position. Do 10 times on each side.

For any exercise that requires kneeling, sitting, or lying on the floor, do the exercise on a mat, a thick carpet, or a folded towel.

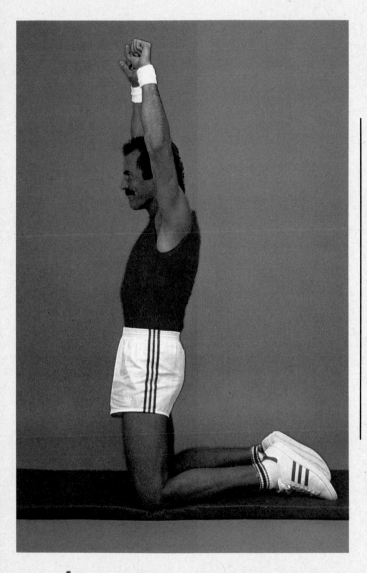

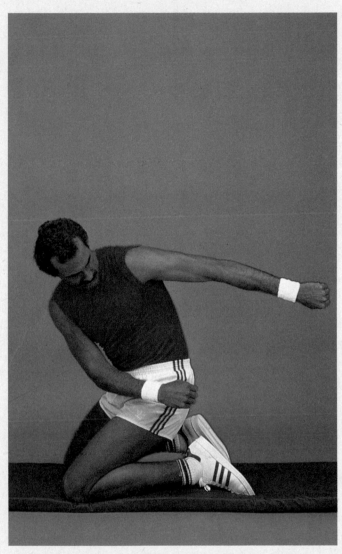

1 Kneel with the legs together, arms overhead, hands in fists.

2 Swing both arms down to the left side, sitting back on the heels at the same time. Return to the starting position, and repeat to the right side. Do 16 to 20 times, alternating left and right.

Do this movement sharply, like the stroke in paddling a canoe.

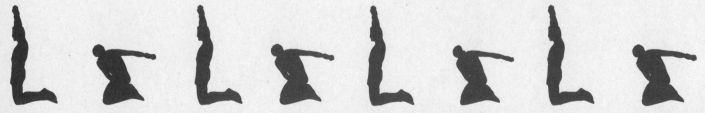

LIFT-OFF

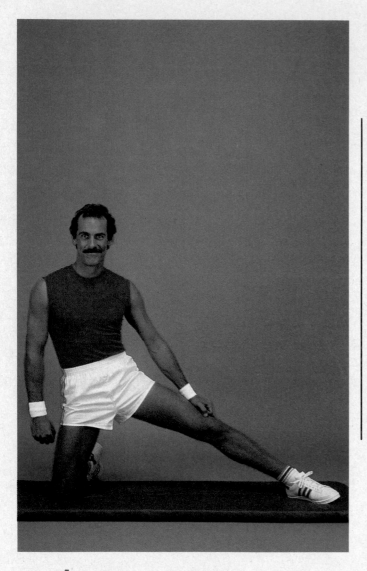

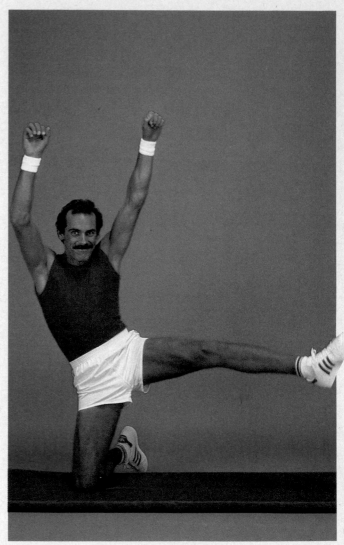

1 Kneel on the right knee, left leg straight to the side, arms at the sides.

2 Swing both arms up, and lift the left leg. Return to the starting position. Do 8 times with each leg.

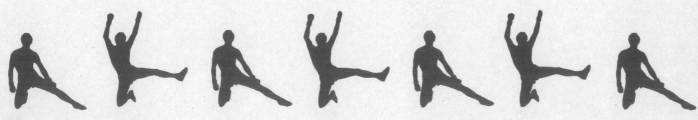

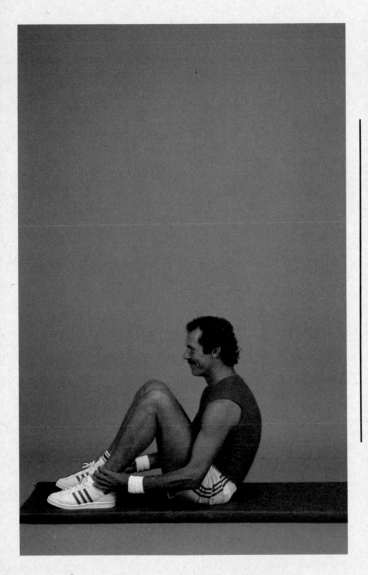

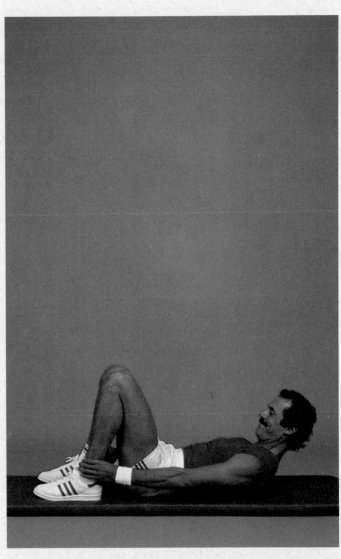

1 Sit with the knees bent, feet wide apart, heels close to the hips, hands holding the ankles.

2 Keeping the hands on the ankles and the feet on the floor, lower the back to the floor, but keep the head up off the floor. Still maintaining the foot and hand positions, sit up. Do 10 times.

PRESS IT

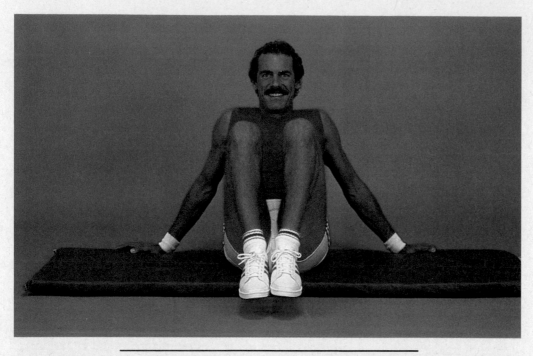

1 Sit with the hands on the floor, knees bent to the chest, feet off the floor.

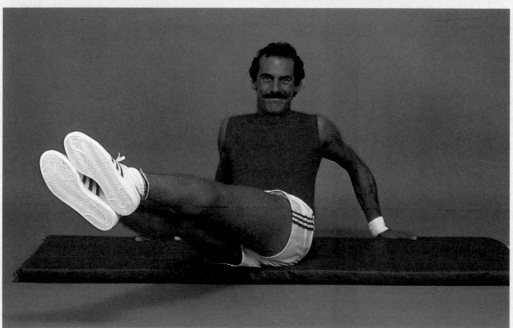

2 Extend both legs to the right. Bend the knees back toward the chest, and then extend the legs to the left. Do 15 to 20 times, alternating right and left.

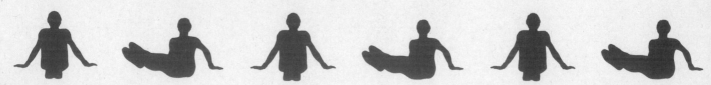

1 Sit on the floor with the feet wide apart, arms out to the sides.

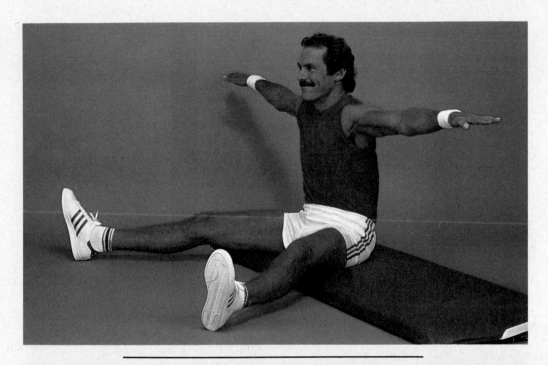

2 Touch the left hand to the right foot. Return to the starting position. Then touch the right hand to the left foot. Do 20 times, alternating left and right.

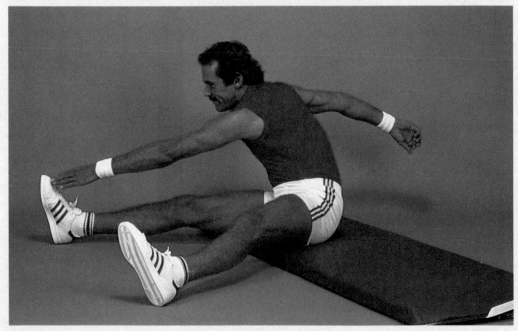

PULL-UP

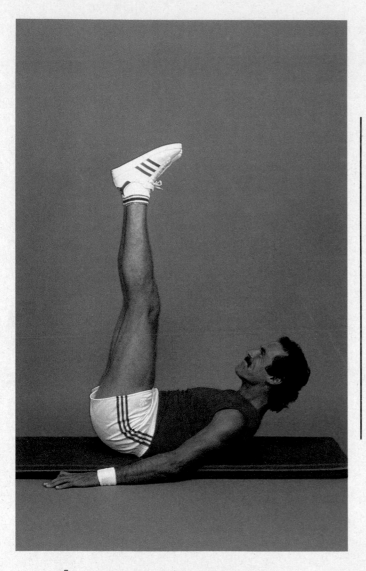

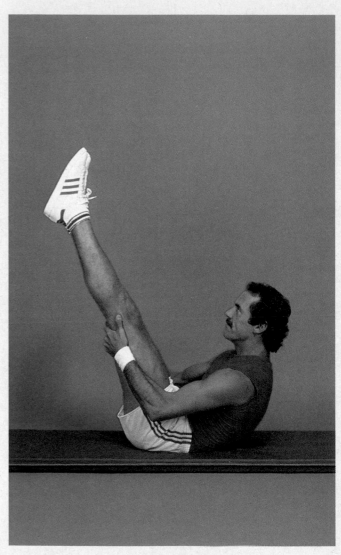

1 Lie on the back with both legs extended up, arms at the sides. The head may be up off the floor or resting on the floor—whichever feels more comfortable for the back.

2 Raise the torso off the floor, and grip the legs as high up as possible. Hold. Return to the starting position. Do 8 times.

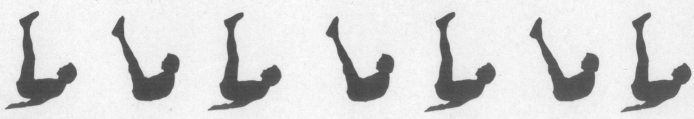

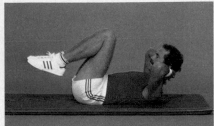

1 Lie on the back with the hands clasped behind the head, knees bent in toward the chest. The head may be up off the floor or resting on the floor—whichever feels more comfortable for the back.

2 Extend both legs straight up.

3 Bend the knees back in toward the chest. Then extend the legs forward. Bring the knees back in toward the chest again. Do 8 times, alternately extending the legs up and then forward.

Extend the legs forward at an angle that is comfortable for the back—one that contracts the stomach muscles but does not stress the back.

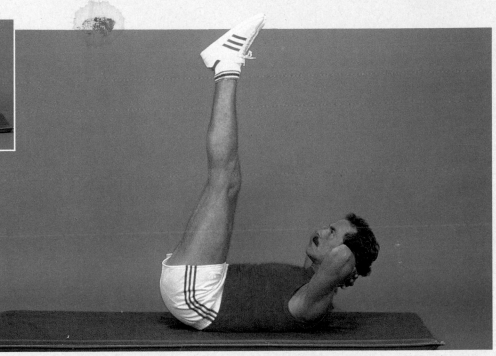

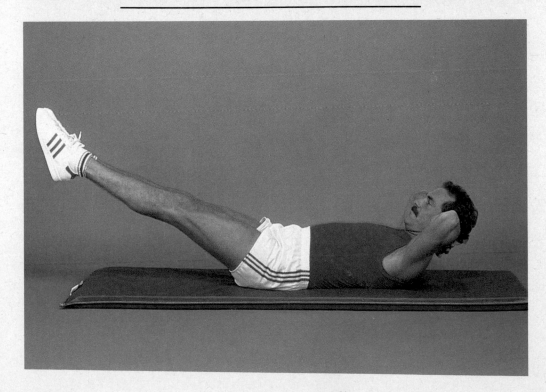

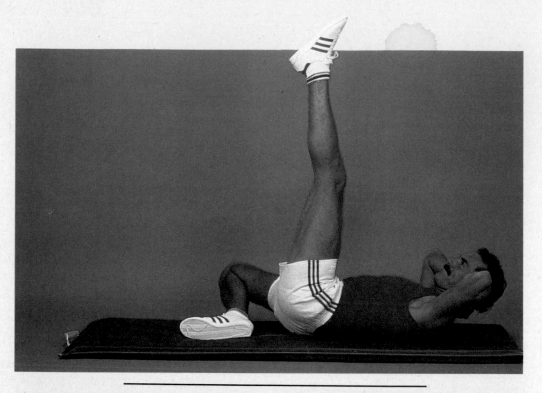

1 Lie on the back, right knee bent so that the foot is turned in toward the body, left leg straight up. Clasp the hands behind the head. The head may be up off the floor or resting on the floor—whichever feels more comfortable for the back.

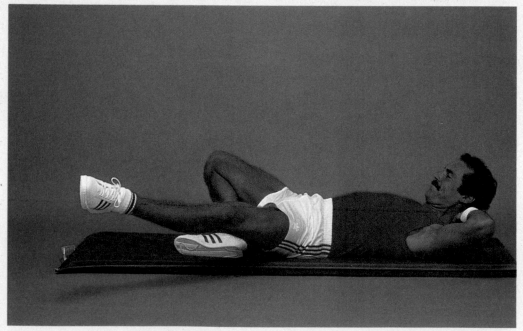

2 Lower the left leg to the side as far as possible. Return the leg up to the starting position. Do 8 times with each leg.

FLY OVER

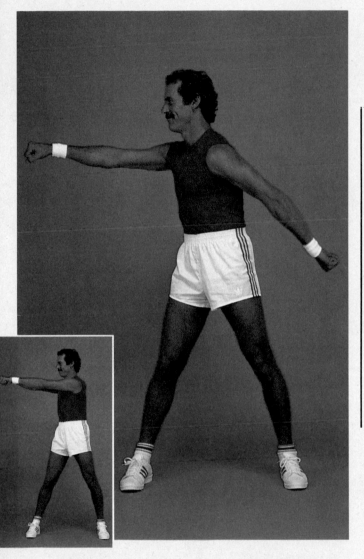

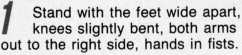

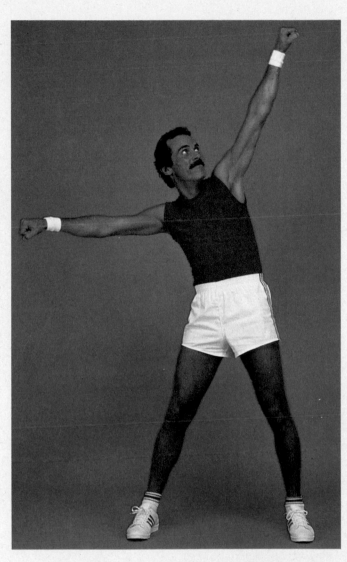

1 Stand with the feet wide apart, knees slightly bent, both arms out to the right side, hands in fists.

2 Circle the left arm down and to the left.

3 Continue in a circular motion, swinging the arm up overhead and down again to meet the right arm. Circle the left arm 15 times. Then starting with both arms out to the left side, circle the right arm 15 times.

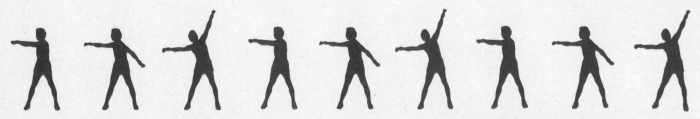

REACH
AND SINK

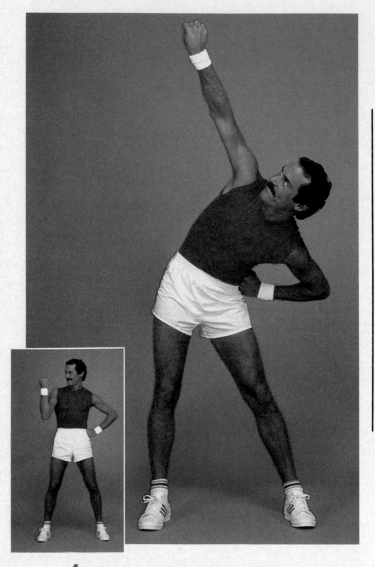

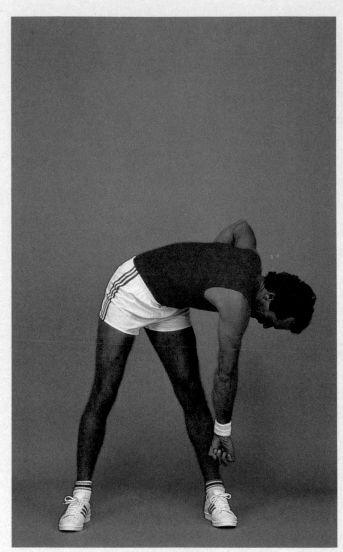

1 Stand with the feet wide apart, knees slightly bent, left hand on the hip, right arm bent up at the side with the hand in a fist.

2 Twist the right arm up so that the palm faces back, while leaning the body to the left.

3 Then bend the arm in to the starting position, and twist the arm down to the left side so that the palm faces forward. Return to the starting position. Do 10 times with each arm.

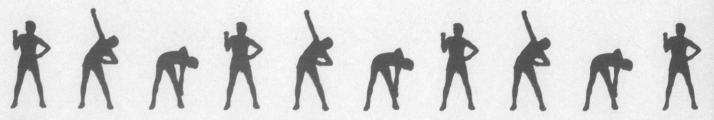

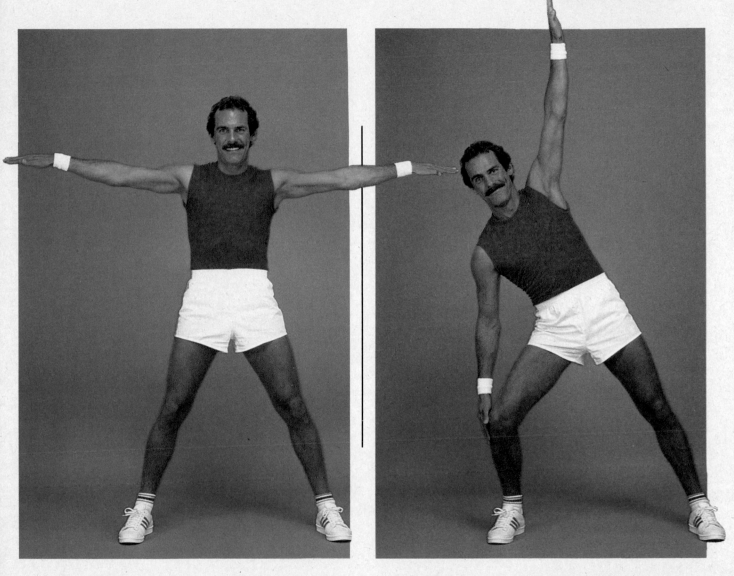

1 Stand with the feet wide apart, knees slightly bent, arms out to the sides.

2 Bend the right knee, and lean to the right. Touch the right hand to the right knee, and raise the left hand straight up. Repeat to the left. Do 15 times, alternating right and left.

Great for the arms and legs, as well as the waistline.

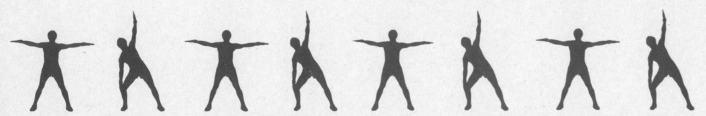

GOOD TURNOUT

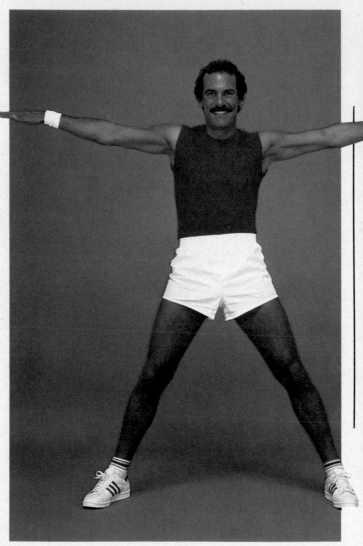

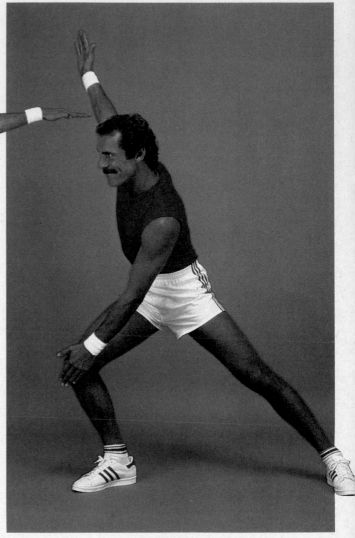

1 Stand with the feet wide apart, knees slightly bent, arms out to the sides.

2 Bend the right knee, turn to the right slightly, and touch the left hand to the right knee. Return to the starting position. Then touch the right hand to the left knee. Do 10 times, alternating right and left.

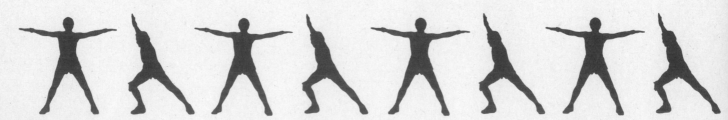

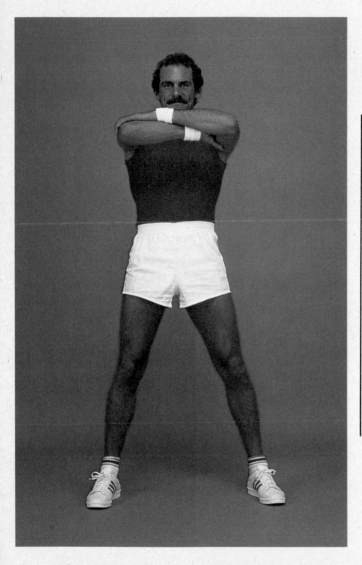

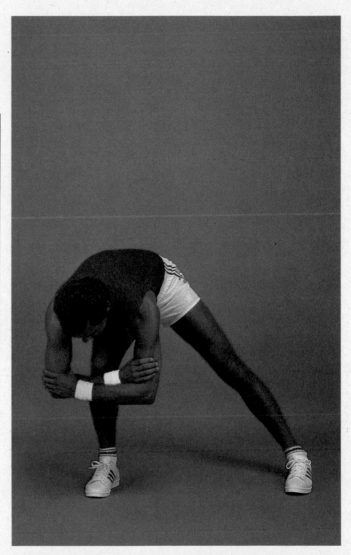

1 Stand with the feet wide apart, hands holding the elbows.

2 Bend the torso over the floor, bend the right knee, and swing both arms to the right leg below the knee. Return to the starting position. Then swing the arms down to the left leg. Do 15 times, alternating right and left.

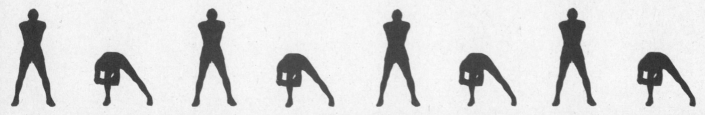

HURDLER'S MOVE

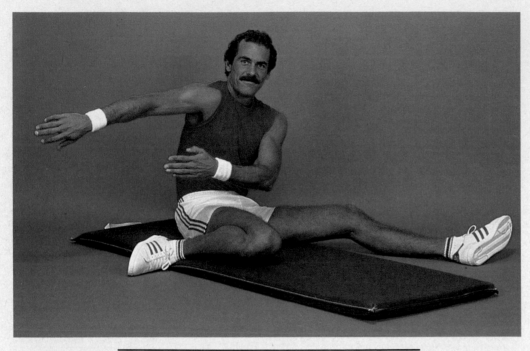

1 Sit in a hurdler's position with the right leg bent back, left leg extended to the side, both arms extended to the right side.

If you have weak knees, bend the leg in front of the body, not in back.

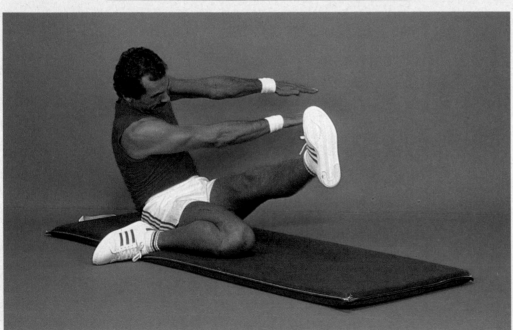

2 Raise the left leg and swing it to the right. At the same time, swing both arms to the left. Return to the starting position. Do 10 times on each side.

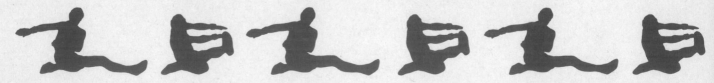

1 Lie on the back with the feet wide apart, hands clasped behind the head, head resting on the floor.

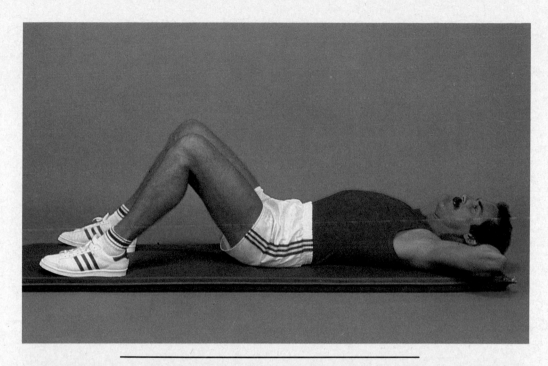

2 Pull the head and shoulders up, try to touch the elbows together, and press the lower back into the floor. Hold for 5 counts. Return to the starting position. Do 10 times.

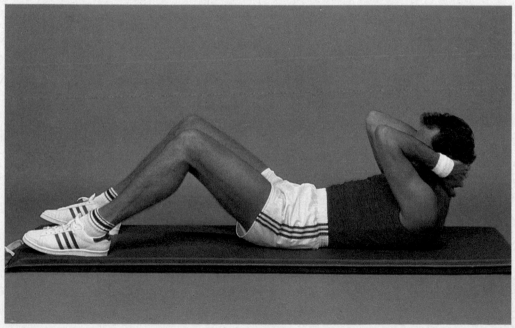

CURL UP

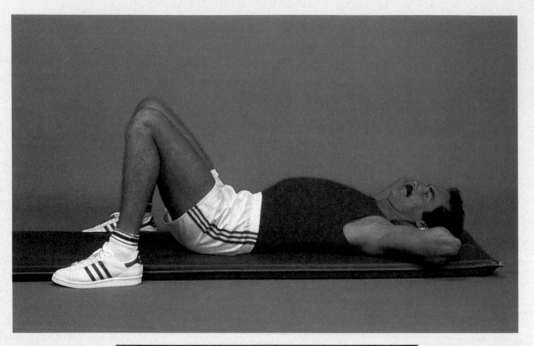

1 Lie on the back with the feet wide apart, heels close to the hips, hands clasped behind the head. The head may be up off the floor or resting on the floor— whichever feels more comfortable for the back.

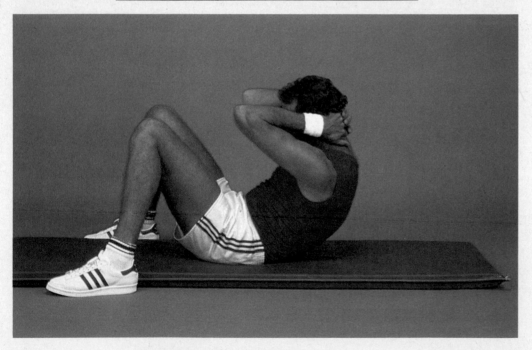

2 Keeping the feet in position on the floor, sit up as far as possible. Return to the starting position. Do 10 times.

1 Sit with the feet wide apart on the floor, knees wide, hands on the floor at the hips, hips off the floor.

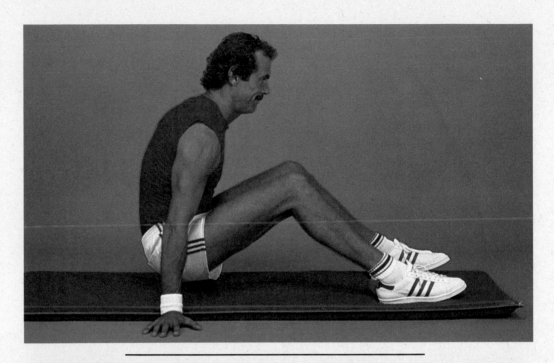

2 Push the hips back behind the hands. Return to the starting position. Do 10 times.

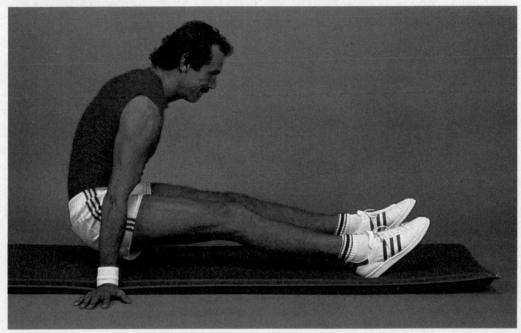

STRENGTHEN THE BACK

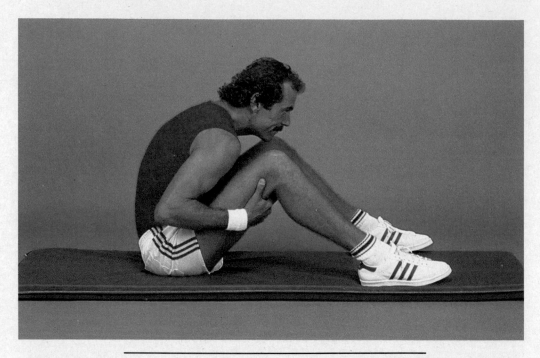

1 Sit on the floor with the knees bent, feet wide apart and flat on the floor, hands holding the legs behind the knees, chest close to the legs.

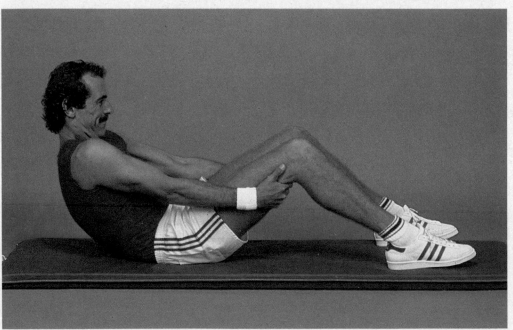

2 Keeping the back rounded, slowly lower the back by straightening the arms. Do not lower any farther than the position with straight arms. Return to the starting position. Do 10 times.

Excellent for strengthening the stomach and back muscles.

1 Sit with the knees bent, feet crossed, arms extended to the right.

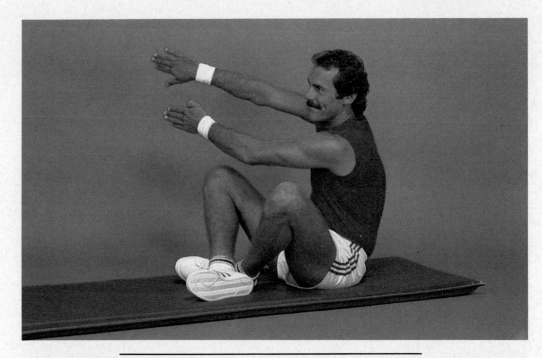

2 Extend the right leg to the side. At the same time, swing the arms to the left. Return to the starting position. Do 10 times on each side.

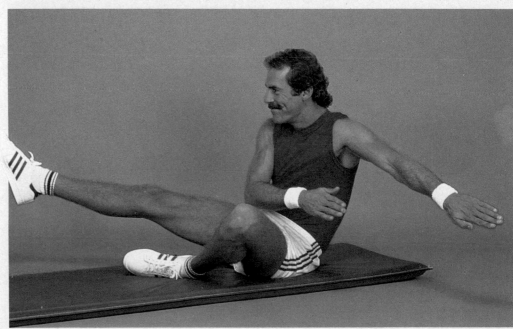

BODY
CONTROL

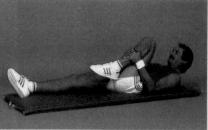

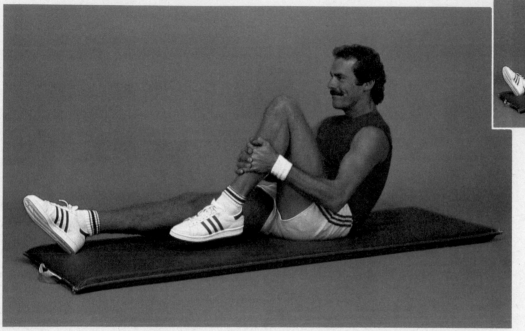

1 Lie on the back, right leg extended on the floor, left knee bent in toward the chest, hands holding the knee, head and shoulders up off the floor.

2 Holding the knee, sit up.

3 Then extend the left leg forward, and swing the arms out to the sides. Bend the knee, grip it, and return to the starting position. Do 10 times with each leg.

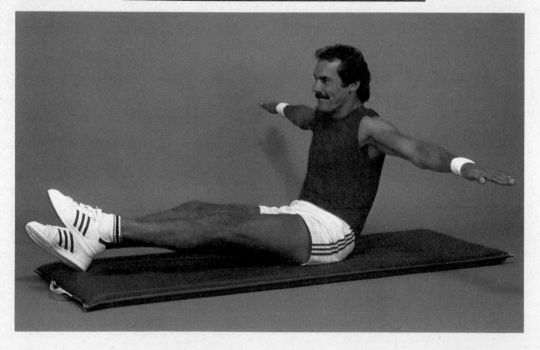

1 Lie on the right side, weight on the right elbow and left hand.

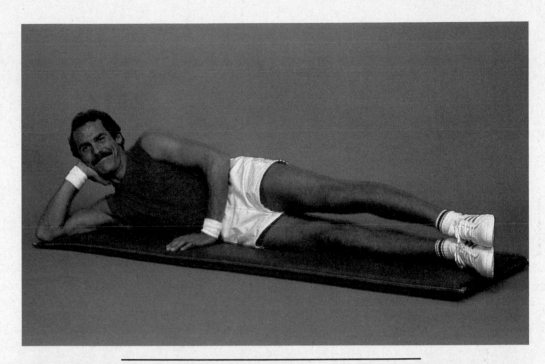

2 Lift both legs up off the floor. Bring the legs forward until they are at a right angle to the body, and lower them to the floor. Lift the legs and return them to the starting position. Do 10 times on each side.

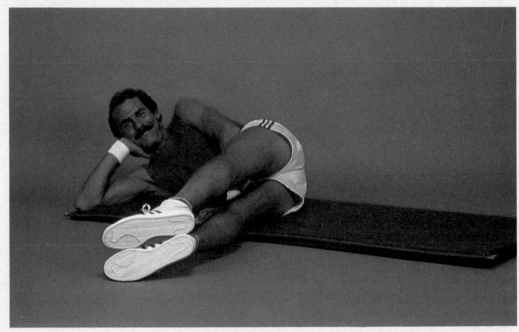

POWER LIFT

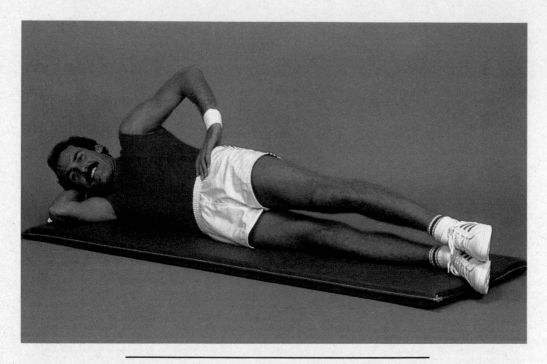

1 Lie on the right side on the floor, legs extended, head on the right arm, left hand on the hip.

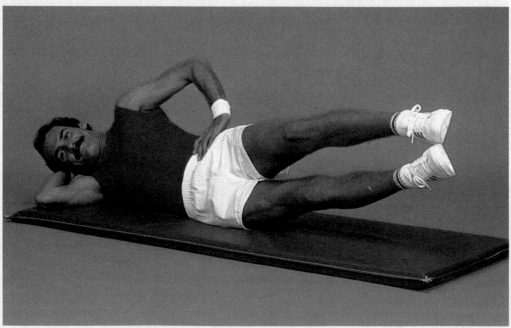

2 Raise both legs up as high as possible. Lower the legs to the floor. Do 10 times on each side.

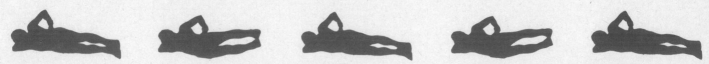

1 Sit on the floor with the knees bent, weight on the heels, hands in fists at the ankles.

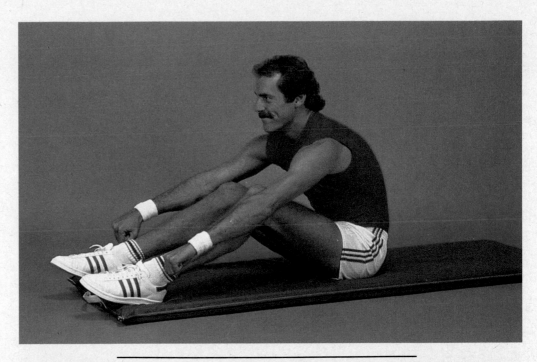

2 Pull the arms back toward the chest and straighten the knees, as if you were rowing a boat. Return to the starting position. Continue for 20 strokes.

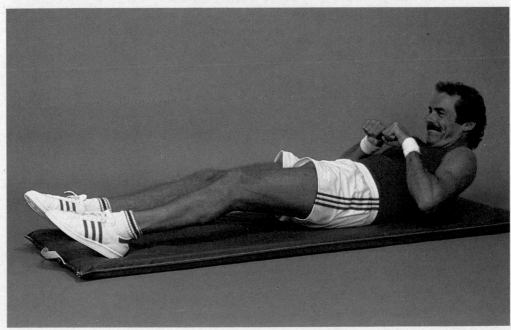

ADVANCED PROGRAM

REACH FOR IT

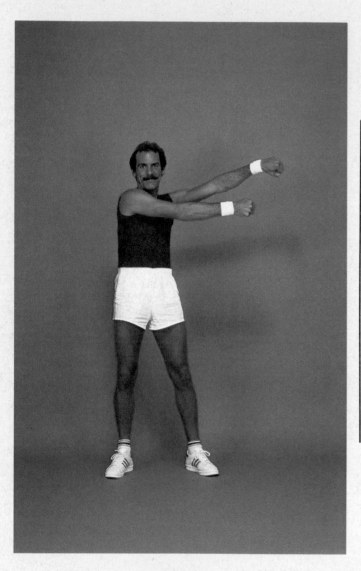

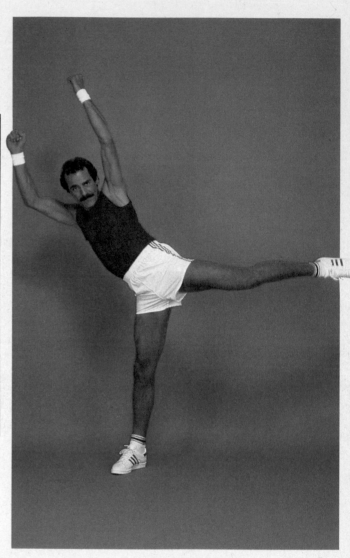

1 Stand with the feet wide apart, arms extended to the left side.

2 Swing both arms overhead to the right, lean the torso to the right, and raise the left leg up. Return to the starting position. Do 10 times to each side.

Work on that waistline!

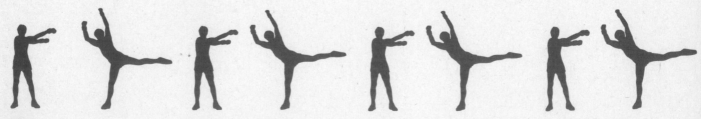

SWING IT

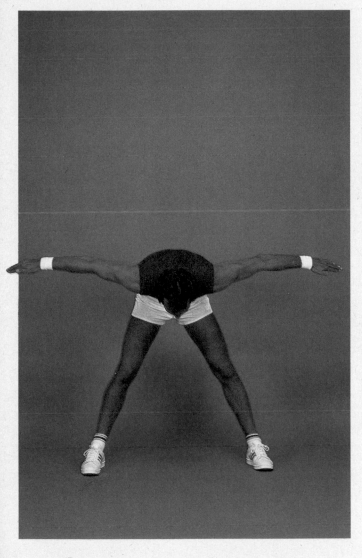

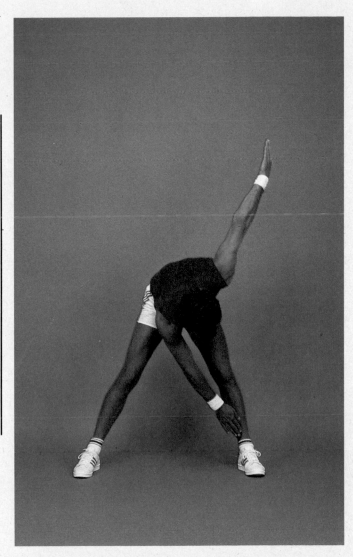

1 Stand with the torso bent over the floor, knees slightly bent, arms out to the sides.

2 Touch the right hand to the left ankle, then the left hand to the right ankle. Do 10 to 15 times, alternating right and left.

This exercise helps get rid of overhang at the belt and sides.

SIDE
WINDUP

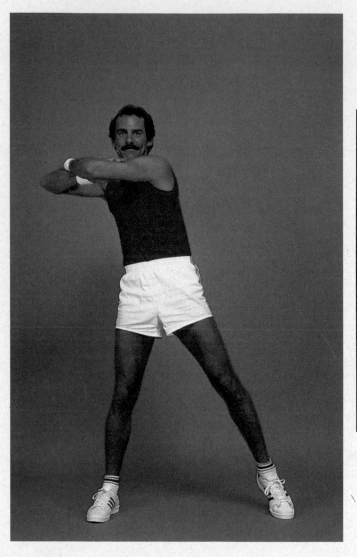 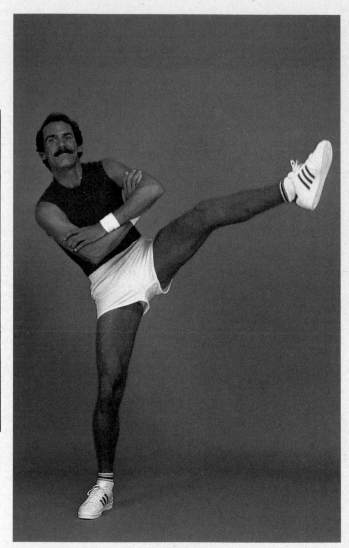

1 Stand with the weight on the right leg, left leg to the side with the weight on the toes, arms to the right side with the hands holding the elbows.

2 Raise the left leg up to the side as high as possible, and swing the arms (in the folded position) toward the left leg. Return to the starting position. Do 8 times with each leg.

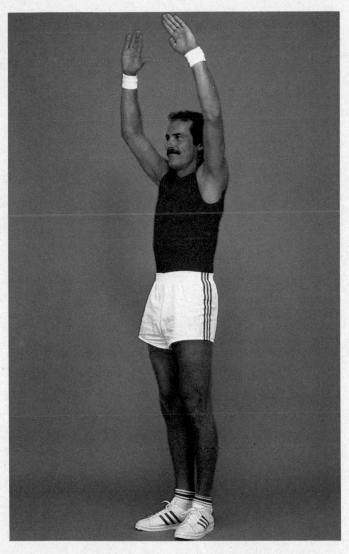

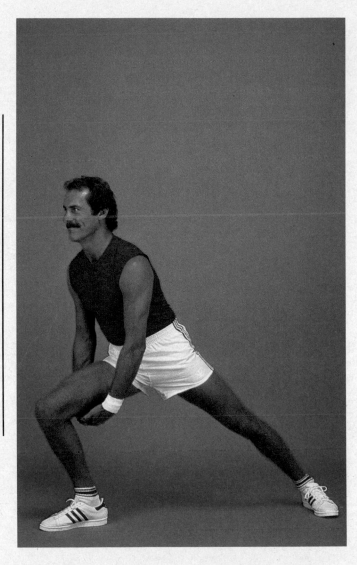

1 Stand with the feet together, arms extended overhead.

2 Lunge forward with the right leg, and touch the hands together behind the right thigh. Return to the starting position. Do 8 times with each leg.

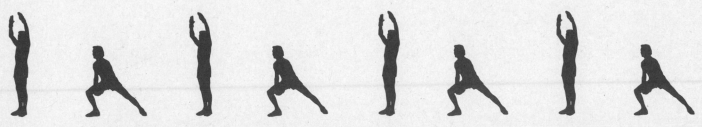

STRONG NOW

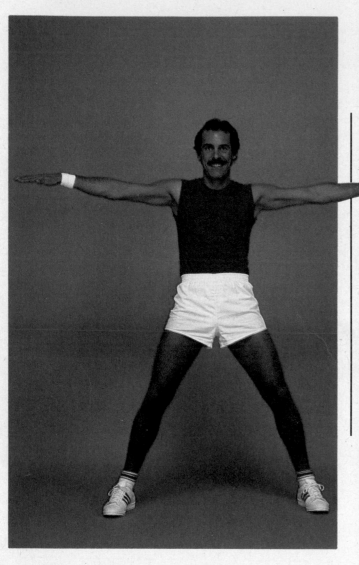 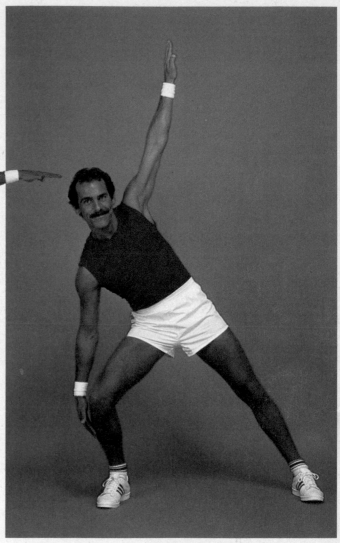

1 Stand with the feet wide apart, knees slightly bent, arms out to the sides.

2 Bend the right knee, lean to the right, touch the right hand to the right calf, and raise the left hand straight up. Repeat to the left side. Do 15 times, alternating right and left.

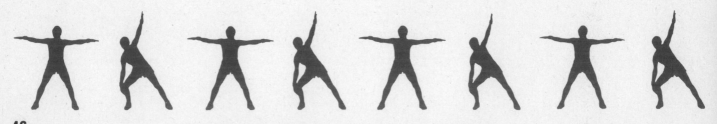

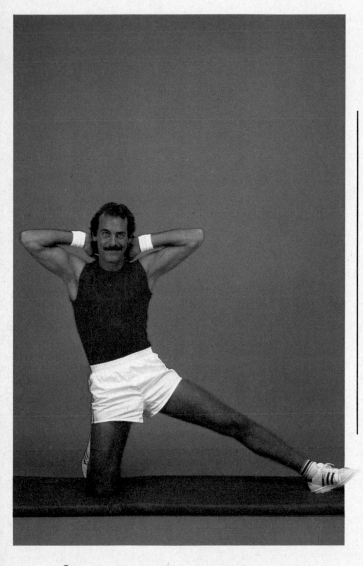

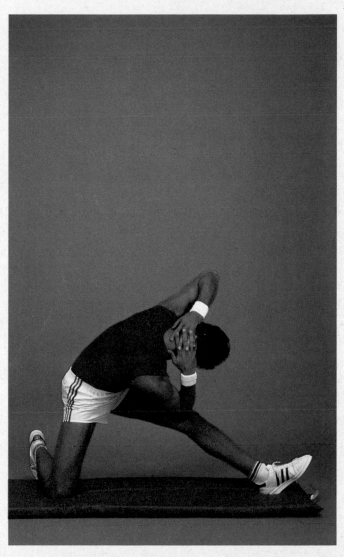

1 Kneel on the right knee, left leg extended to the side, hands behind the head.

2 Twist and touch the right elbow to the left knee. Return to the starting position. Do 8 times on each side.

BIG TWIST

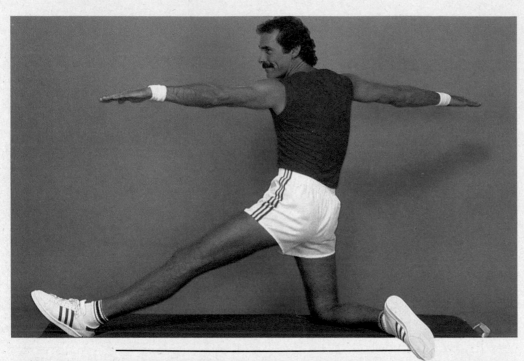

1 Kneel on the right knee, left leg extended to the side, arms extended out to the sides.

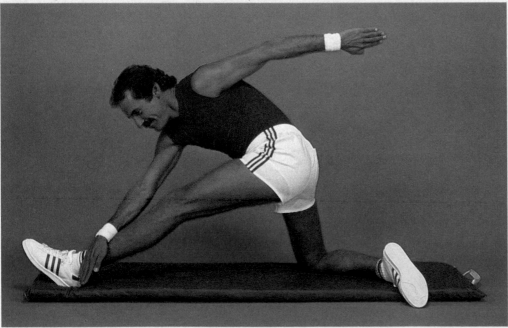

2 Twist and try to touch the right hand to the floor outside the left ankle. Return to the starting position. Do 8 times on each side.

Guaranteed to firm the waistline.

1 Sit with the weight on the elbows, both legs extended directly to the right side.

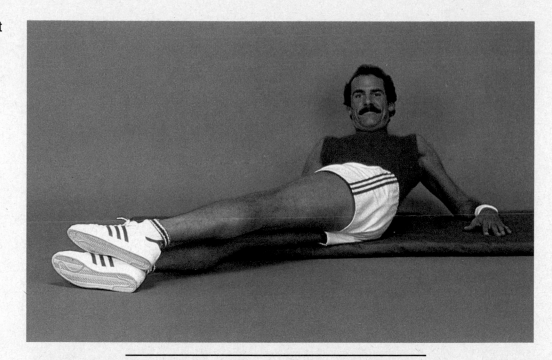

2 Lift both legs and move them in an arc up, over, and down to the floor on the left side. Then arc the legs up and over to the right side to return to the starting position. Do 20 times.

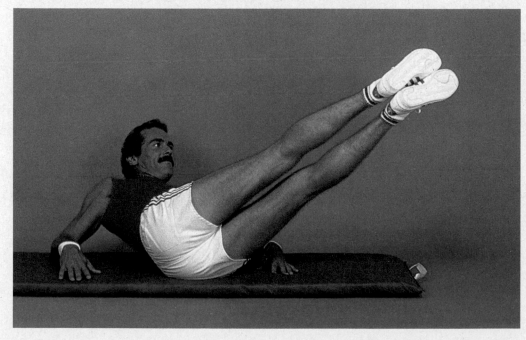

SUPER PRESS

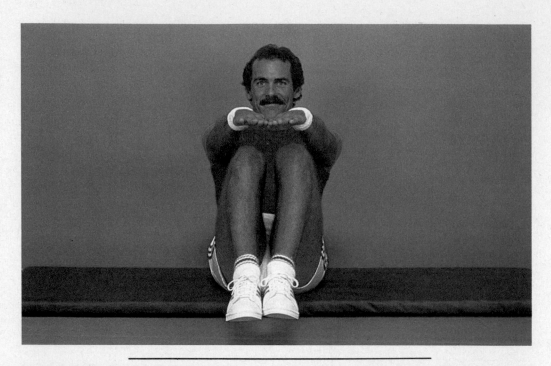

1 Sit with the knees bent, feet off the floor, arms extended straight forward.

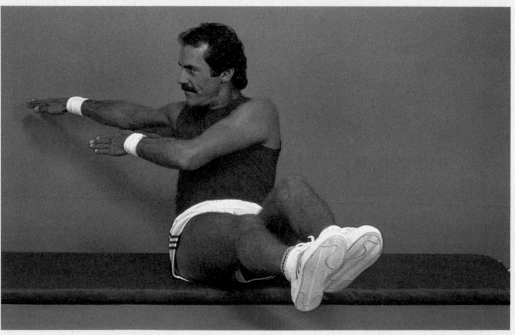

2 Extend both legs to the left side. At the same time, press both arms to the right. Return to the starting position. Then extend the legs to the right, arms to the left. Do 10 to 20 times, alternating left and right.

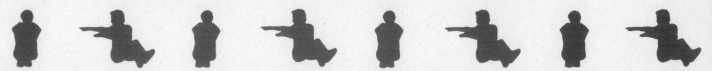

1 Sit with the feet on the floor, knees bent, hands behind the head.

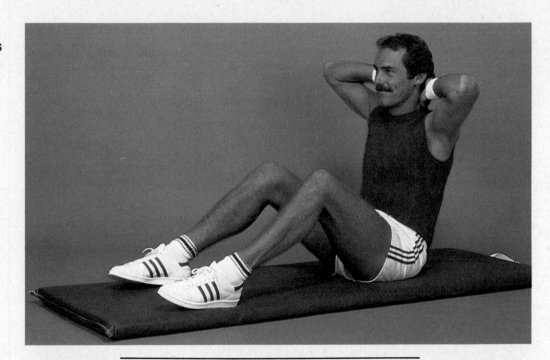

2 Bend the left knee in toward the chest, and touch the right elbow to the knee. At the same time, kick the right leg out. Then bring in the right knee to touch the left elbow, and kick out the left leg. Do 10 to 15 times, alternating left and right.

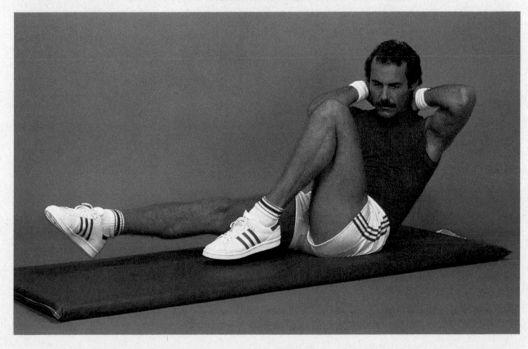

POWER SIT

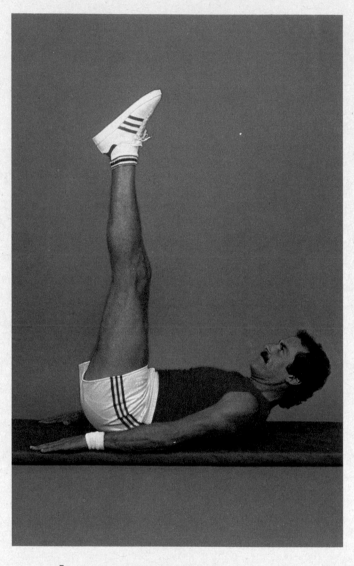

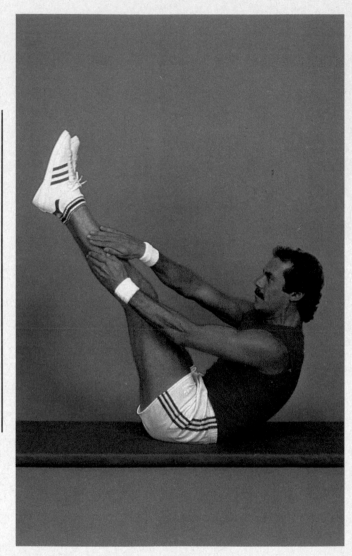

1 Lie on the back with the legs up, arms at the sides, head up off the floor.

2 Raise the head and torso off the floor, and grab the outside of the left leg with both hands. Return to the starting position. Repeat, grabbing the outside of the right leg. Do 8 times, alternating to the left and right.

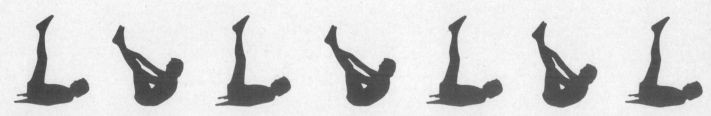

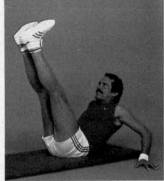

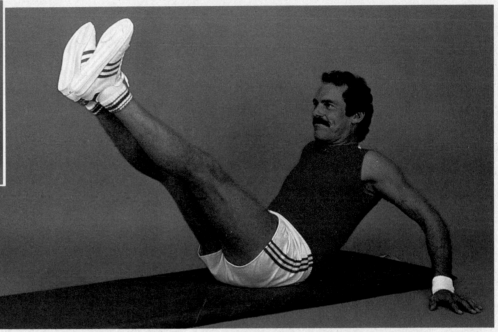

1 Sit with the weight on the hands, legs extended up, toes turned out to the sides.

2 Lower both legs slightly. Then return the legs to the straight up position. Do 4 times.

3 Then sit up and round the back. Return to the starting position, and lower the legs 4 more times.

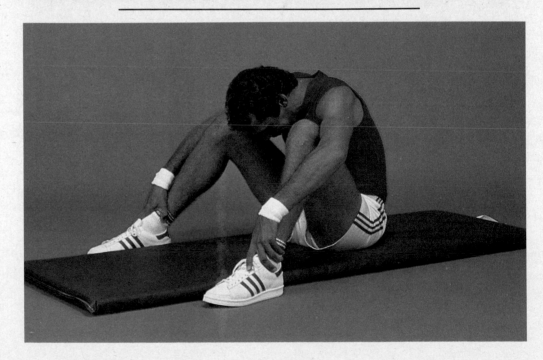

THE STRENGTHENER

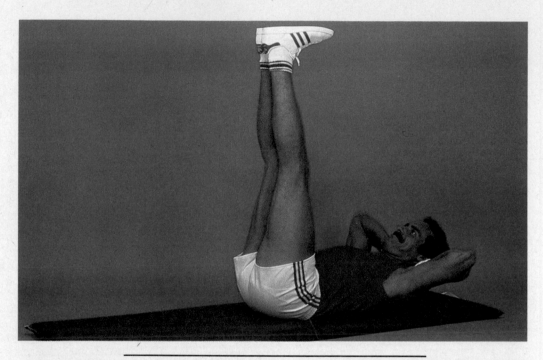

1 Lie on the back with the legs extended straight up, feet flat, hands clasped behind the head, head up off the floor.

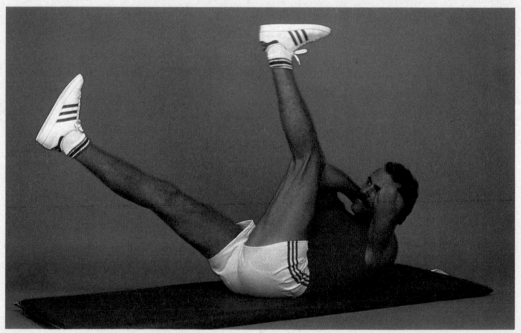

2 Swing the left leg toward the head, and try to touch the right elbow to the left knee. Repeat with the right leg, touching the left elbow to the knee. Do 15 to 20 times, alternating left and right.

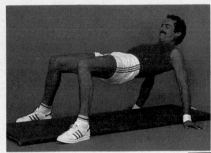

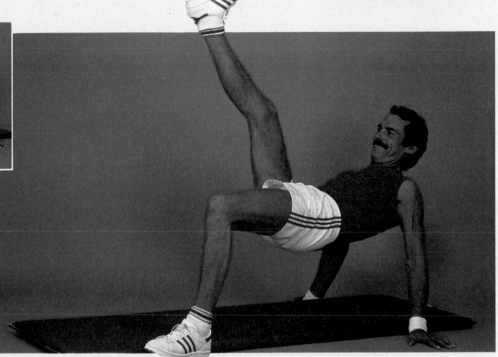

1 Assume a "gymnastic table" position, with the weight on the hands and feet, hips up.

2 Extend the right leg straight up and toward the head.

3 Then lower the leg toward the floor, but do not touch it to the floor. Do 8 times with each leg.

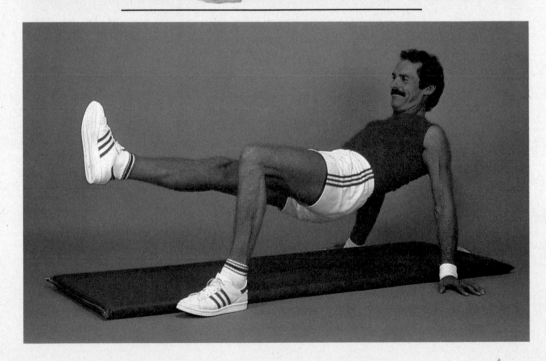

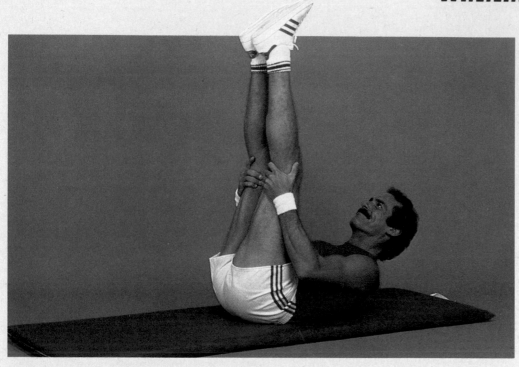

1 Lie on the back with the legs up, hands holding the backs of the legs, head up off the floor.

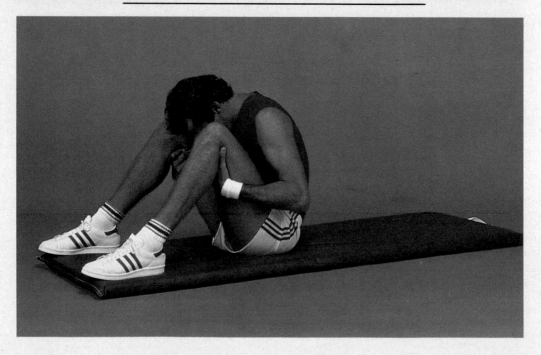

2 Sit up, bend the knees, and place the feet flat on the floor. Open the knees, and press the head down. Return to the starting position. Do 5 times.

CAT ARCH

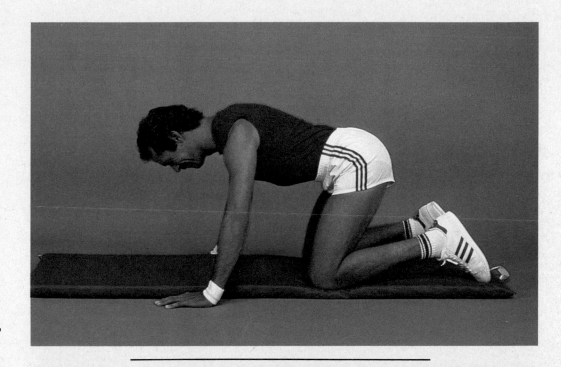

1 Kneel on the hands and knees, head down, back flat.

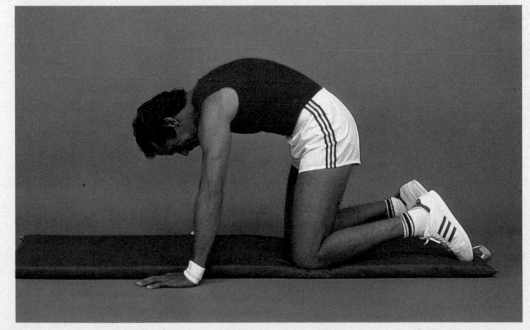

2 Slowly tilt the hips forward, round the back up as high as possible, and pull in the stomach muscles. Hold this position for 5 counts. Return to the starting position. Do 5 times.

This exercise strengthens the back and stomach muscles.

THE KICKER

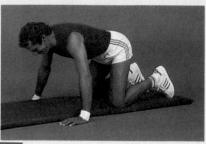

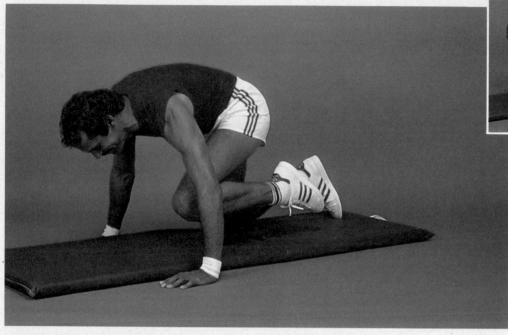

1 Kneel on the hands and knees, head down, back flat.

2 Bend the left knee in toward the chest as far as possible.

3 Then extend the leg back, bending the knee so that the lower leg is up. Return to the starting position. Do 8 times with each leg.

This exercise strengthens the back and helps eliminate bloating in the stomach area.

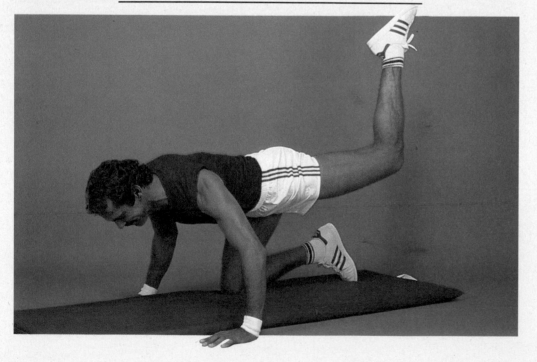

1 Lie on the back with the legs extended, arms at the sides, head on the floor.

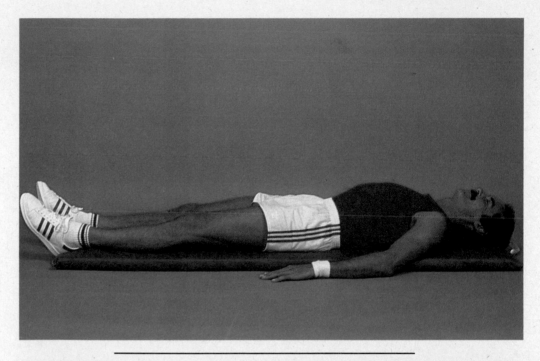

2 Slowly pull the right knee toward the chest, grasping it with both hands. At the same time, lift the head and press the nose to the knee. Hold for 5 counts. Return to the starting position. Do 5 times with each leg.

This exercise relieves stress on the back and neck.

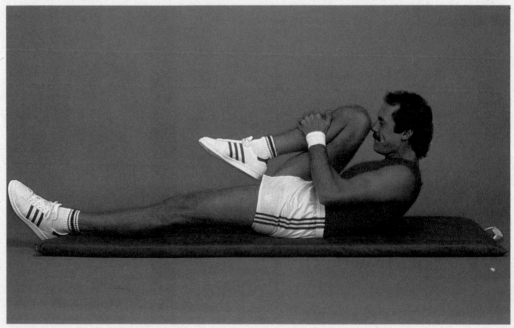

SCISSORS

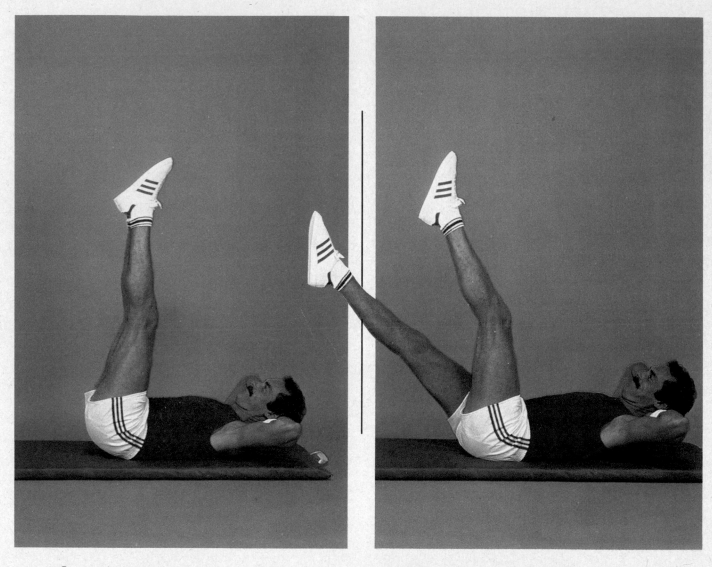

1 Lie on the back with the legs extended up, hands clasped behind the head. The head may be up off the floor or resting on the floor—whichever feels more comfortable for the back.

2 Alternately swing the legs forward and back, like a scissors kick, for 10 to 20 counts.

This exercise helps return circulation to the pre-exercise state and helps prevent pooling of blood in the legs.

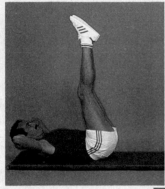

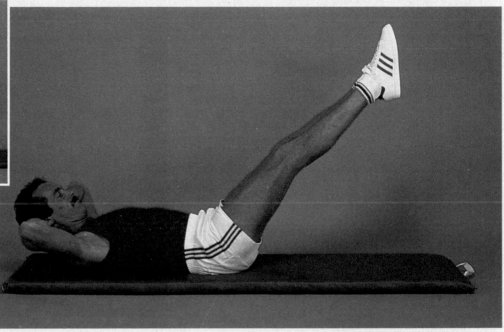

1 Lie on the back with the legs extended straight up, hands clasped under the head. The head may be up off the floor or resting on the floor—whichever feels more comfortable for the back.

2 Press the back into the floor, and slowly lower both legs to the floor.

3 Bend the knees in toward the chest. Then extend the legs up again to the starting position. Do 5 to 8 times.

This exercise strengthens the back and lengthens the stomach muscles to prevent bulging.

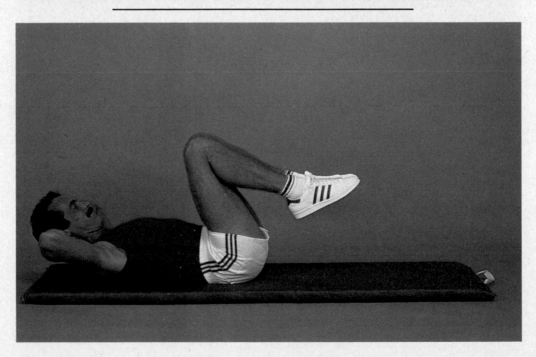

BICYCLE

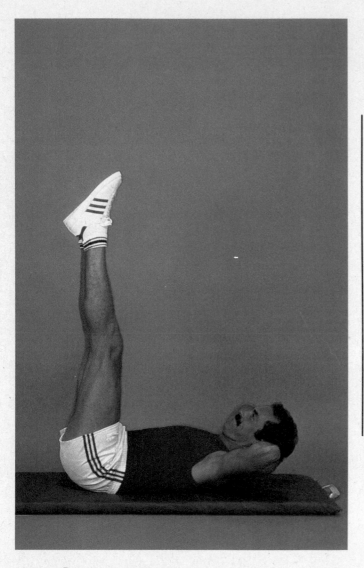

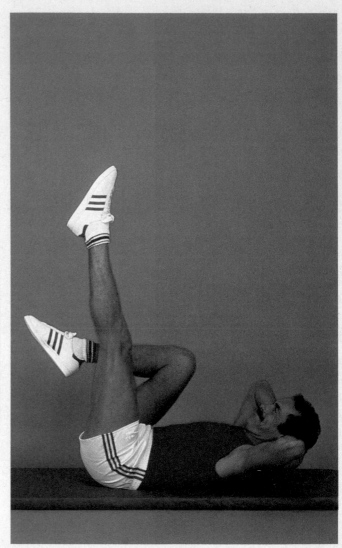

1 Lie on the back with the legs extended straight up, hands clasped under the head. The head may be up off the floor or resting on the floor—whichever feels more comfortable for the back.

2 "Bicycle" the legs in long stretches out, alternating left and right, for 20 to 30 counts.

1 Kneel on the hands and knees, toes curled to rest on the floor.

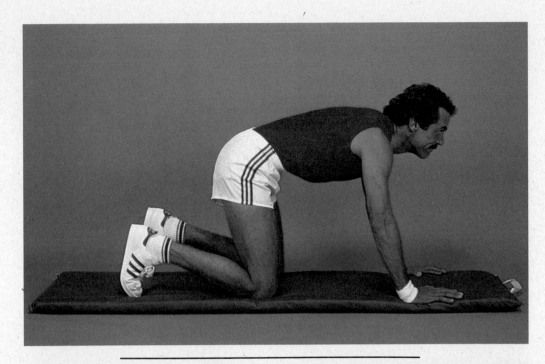

2 Lift the hips, straighten the legs, and arch the back up. Pull in the stomach muscles, and try to press the heels back toward the floor. Feel every muscle and ligament being stretched and tightened. Hold for 5 counts. Return to the starting position. Do 5 times.

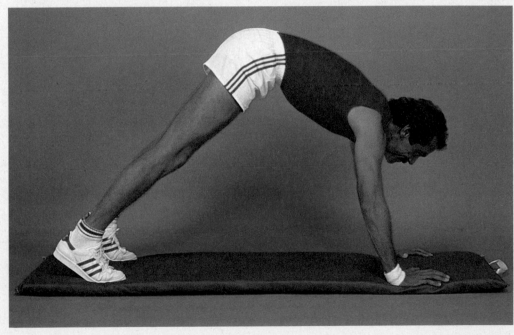

REV UP

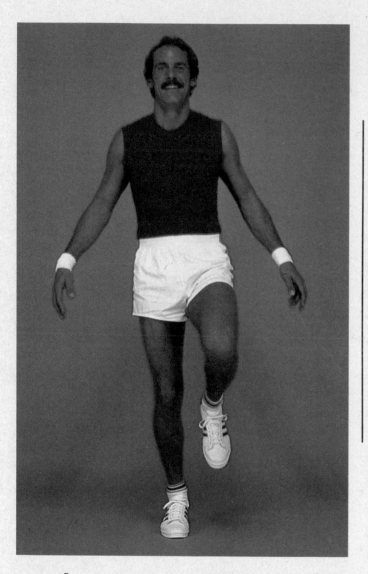

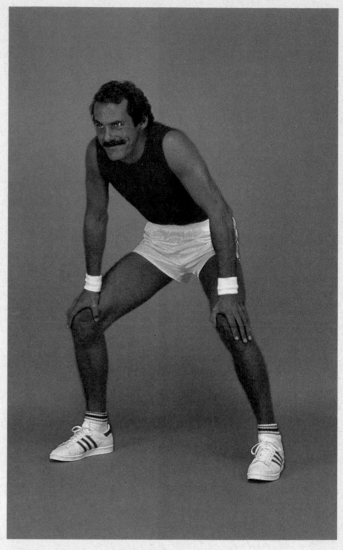

1 Run at a very slow pace, shaking the arms at the sides. Start with 1 minute, and advance gradually to 3 minutes.

2 Stand with the feet wide apart, knees bent, hands on the knees. Lift the shoulders, and hold for 5 counts. Lower the shoulders. Do 3 times.

This exercise restores the body and raises the energy level. You should feel relaxed and invigorated.

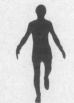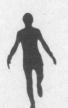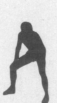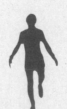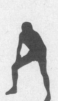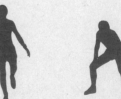

NOW AVAILABLE ON VIDEOTAPE

FLATTEN YOUR STOMACH

YES! For only $19.95 you can enjoy exercising your way to a slimmer, firmer waistline with this new video from Consumer Guide®. You just put the videocassette in your VCR, start it up and follow the exercise instructor on your TV screen.

Everything you'll be doing is based on the best-selling Consumer Guide® "Flatten Your Stomach" books. You'll do:

Warm-ups to stretch and relax your body

A balanced set of exercises to tone and firm all four major abdominal muscles

Cool downs to help you avoid soreness

Exercises especially created for men only

By using this video you can see exactly how each exercise is done. Once you've got the hang of it, use your videocassette each time you exercise to keep on track and work out at the right pace.

Isn't it worth it to invest in the figure you've always wanted? If you're not completely satisfied with this videocassette, we'll take it back and send you a full refund. You've got nothing to lose but some inches on your waistline.

So put your order in the mail today!

ONLY $19.95

NEW·QUICK·WAY TO
FLATTEN YOUR STOMACH
FOR MEN ONLY

CONSUMER GUIDE®
HOME VIDEO

RUNNING TIME: 30 MINUTES

FOR MEN ONLY